Coping with Chronic Obstructive Pulmonary Disease

Also by Elaine Fantle Shimberg

Coping with Chronic Heartburn

How to Get Out of the Hospital Alive (coauthor)

Living with Tourette Syndrome

Depression: What Families Should Know

Strokes: What Families Should Know

Relief from IBS: Irritable Bowel Syndrome

Gifts of Time (coauthor)

Coping with

Chronic

Obstructive

Pulmonary

Disease

Elaine Fantle Shimberg

St. Martin's Griffin ✦ New York

Material in Chapter Four, "What Caregivers Need to Know," is adapted from Jo-Von Tucker, COPD patient, in *Courage and Information for Life with Chronic Obstructive Pulmonary Disease,* by Rick Carter, Ph.D., Brooke Nicotra, M.D., and Jo-Von Tucker. New Technology Publishing. Onset, MA, 2001

www.stmartins.com

Library of Congress Cataloging-in-Publication Data

Shimberg, Elaine Fantle, 1937–
        Coping with COPD / Elaine Fantle Shimberg.— 1st ed.
            p. cm.
        Includes bibliography references (p. 223) and index.
        ISBN 0-312-30777-2
        1. Lungs—Diseases, Obstructive. I. Title: Coping with chronic obstructive pulmonary disease. II. Title.

RC776.O3S526 2003
616.2'4—dc21

                                                                                        2003046880

First Edition: October 2003

10   9   8   7   6   5   4   3   2   1

Dedicated to

Jo-Von Tucker

For her courage, caring, and cooperation

Contents

Author's Note

The information contained in this book is based on the author's research and is intended to help you better understand chronic obstructive pulmonary disease and how it affects patients and their families. It is in no way meant to replace advice by a qualified medical professional. Medical opinions specific to you as an individual can be given only by a physician who has examined you and is aware of your unique medical history and physical condition.

Never self-diagnose. Always seek help from a qualified physician.

Acknowledgments

There are many voices represented in this book. Some are those of medical professionals who have devoted their careers to working with patients who have COPD, while others are those who have "walked the walk," people with COPD and those who love them.

Many thanks to all who shared their thoughts and expertise, both lay and professional experts: Jeff Mador, M.D.; Susan A. Ward; Jo-Von Tucker; Mark Vaaler, M.D.; Lee Kirkman, M.D.; Dorothy Robertson; Ted Fall; Genevieve Cusick; Paul Foynes; Ann Shedd; Francis Birch; Mickey Weill; Kathryn Smith; Mary Burns, R.N.; Richard Casaburi, Ph.D., M.D.; Jane H. Wad; Gail O. French; Steve Wilson, Ph.D.; Richard F. Lockey, M.D.; Kim Lebowitz, Ph.D.; Saadia Greenberg of the Administration on Aging; Patricia Underwood; "PJ"; DeeDee Brayboy; Shawna Crew; "Vaughn Devon"; and Thomas L. Petty, M.D.

I'd be lost without the research help given to me by Rose Bland and the rest of the staff of the Health Sciences Library at the University of South Florida, so thanks, gang.

I especially appreciate the efforts of three physicians: Lee Kirkman, Mark Vaaler, and Thomas L. Petty. Each of these men gave a most valued commodity—time—to review my manuscript for accuracy. Any errors that may still exist fall upon my shoulders alone.

As always, I thank my funny and faithful friend and agent, Faith Hamlin, and my editor, Heather Jackson, for their trust in me. A special thanks, as well, to my illustrator, Kathy Taylor Zimmerman, and to Veronica Tillis, for her help in proofreading this manuscript.

Foreword

Although COPD is not yet a household word, it soon will be. COPD is the most rapidly growing health problem in the United States and elsewhere in the world. COPD is the only disease in the top ten that continues to rise. Because of the still high prevalence of smoking and the fact that COPD accelerates with age, we will continue to see the problem advance in the foreseeable future.

Elaine Fantle Shimberg, who has written other excellent books on common medical subjects such as stroke, irritable bowel syndrome, and acid reflux (GERD), has produced a masterpiece in this volume. With clarity of style for patients and their families, she carefully explains what COPD is and how it is evaluated by doctors and other health care workers. She puts appropriate emphasis on the patient-doctor relationship, which is so critical to the successful management of COPD. COPD patients must understand their disease and the reasons for the uncomfortable symptoms it causes. Knowing how to cope with any chronic illness is key to the solution.

Although COPD cannot be cured, it can be arrested or slowed in its progress. Of greatest importance is that the quality of life of virtually all COPD patients can be greatly improved.

The key to controlling COPD is its early identification. Shimberg rightly emphasizes the new health care initiatives that promote early identification and treatment. These are the National Lung Health Education Program (NLHEP) and the Global Initiative for Lung Disease (GOLD). Both NLHEP and GOLD will help advance knowledge about COPD and its management. Books like *Coping with COPD* will help the patient and the family understand and deal with COPD.

The key admonition I always give my patients with COPD is, "Remember to live." Do not let COPD get in the way of the pursuit of happiness. Remain optimistic and be in control. Shimberg's book will go a long way in promoting this philosophy.

Thomas L. Petty, M.D.
Co-chairman, NLHEP

Introduction

You probably picked up this book because you or someone you care about has been diagnosed with chronic obstructive pulmonary disease. It's more commonly referred to as COPD, although some people call it COLD (chronic obstructive lung disease) or COAD (chronic obstructive airways disease). But with apologies to Shakespeare, a disease by any other name is still a scary disease.

You may still be numb after learning that what you thought was just an irritating cough along with some breathlessness is actually a chronic disease with no cure at the present time. It's a little overwhelming.

If you don't have the disease yourself and need to have some idea of what it is like, take a deep breath and hold it. Then, let just a fraction of the air out and quickly try to take another breath. You can't. Your lungs can't expand enough to make room for more air. But unless this is your reality, happening every day, you can't imagine the panic. When you can't inhale air to fill your lungs and then exhale completely to make room for another breath, it triggers primordial fears of being buried alive. You gasp, strain, and struggle for each breath.

This is the terror for more than 17 million Americans and 44 million people worldwide who suffer from chronic obstructive pulmonary disease, which actually is an umbrella term for a group of respiratory disorders that block and shut down breathing passages. These disorders include emphysema, chronic bronchitis, and, often, asthmatic bronchitis. It's estimated that, because of lack of awareness and education both on the part of those who are afflicted as well as physicians, the number of those actually suffering with COPD far exceeds patients who already have been diagnosed.

The incidence of COPD, which is the fourth leading cause of death in the United States (behind heart disease, cancer, and stroke), is rising. According to the National Lung Health Education Program (NLHEP), in more than 90 percent of cases, the illness is related to smoking. In fact, smokers are ten times more likely than nonsmokers to die of the disease.

But although COPD is a chronic disease, this book is written about hope, not despair. It shows you how to make each day as meaningful and productive as possible, even with COPD. *Coping with COPD* is intended for those who have been diagnosed with the disease as well as for their families, for COPD can and does affect an entire family. The book describes not only what happens to someone with COPD but also how the disease is treated and illustrates what the family and the patient can do to improve day-to-day living with COPD. It explains the importance of exercise, proper nutrition, and improving breathing techniques, where to find help and support, and how to avoid environmental factors that worsen the disease. It also speaks to caregivers,

showing ways for them to relax, be supportive, and conserve
their own strength as they care for a loved one with COPD.

Although COPD cannot be cured at this time, its sufferers
can improve the length and quality of their lives. New treatments
and medications are being developed continually, and let's hope
the many programs to prevent and stop smoking will reduce the
number of new COPD patients being diagnosed annually.

Do not try to diagnose yourself or a loved one from reading
this book alone. The book's purpose is to inform, not to diagnose
or treat. Always seek the help of a qualified medical professional.

PART ONE

———

Understanding and Treating COPD

What Is Chronic Obstructive Pulmonary Disease?

Chronic obstructive pulmonary disease (COPD) is just what it sounds like. It is chronic, which means an ongoing, progressive, and at present, incurable disease. COPD damages the lungs' ability to take in and expel air. By doing so, COPD decreases lung function.

Actually, COPD is an umbrella name for two or more diseases: chronic bronchitis, emphysema, and, sometimes, asthma. Most commonly, however, the two afflicting diseases are emphysema and chronic bronchitis, each with its own set of unique problems and medical treatments. While asthma symptoms can be controlled, COPD is a permanent condition characterized by the creeping and progressive limitation of airflow.

Although COPD affects twice as many Americans as does diabetes, most people, including patients and their families, know little about the disease or have misinformation about it. Easy breathers (that is, those without COPD) who understand that cigarette smoking is the major cause of COPD, often brush off the diagnosis with a curt and nonsympathetic, "Well, if you hadn't smoked, you wouldn't have gotten it," thus adding to the sense of guilt and frustration of COPD patients who, of course, wish they had known just how harmful smoking could be to their lungs. Every COPD patient I interviewed said in some form, "If I had only known then what I know now!"

Chronic obstructive pulmonary disease doesn't just suddenly hit you one day, like a heart attack or a stroke. It is much more insidious, gradually sneaking up on you like a lion stalking a zebra. COPD becomes progressively worse with age. In fact, the majority of patients aren't even aware of any symptoms until they're in their late forties, fifties, or sixties, at which time it's too late to reverse the damage. According to Thomas L. Petty, M.D., co-chairman of the National Lung Health Education Program and professor of medicine at the University of Colorado Health Science Center in Denver, 15 million cases of COPD are undiagnosed, even in patients who are already exhibiting symptoms.

But, as denial is human, many people probably ignore its existence or attribute the signs to another cause. "I'm out of breath because I just climbed the stairs and I'm out of shape," or "I just can't get rid of this smoker's cough. I guess I'll have to stop smoking." Those with bronchitis or asthma downplay their symptoms, considering their coughing or wheezing to be merely a nuisance and seek medical help only when things get "really bad."

Jo-Von Tucker, who was diagnosed with COPD fifteen years ago, knows this firsthand. In an E-mail interview, she said, "At first I experienced shortness of breath upon exertion, eventually with some chest pain. I had quit smoking (after thirty years of smoking 1½ packs a day) two years before I had any symptoms at all. I assumed, at first, that the shortness of breath was due to the fact that I had gained weight after I quit smoking. But I was plagued with multiple bouts of bronchitis, and eventually a case of pneumonia that nearly killed me."

Tucker said that it wasn't until the doctor gave her the diagnosis of COPD that she realized she had something serious, something that wasn't just going to go away.

COPD IS A SERIOUS DISEASE

COPD is often known as the "silent disease" because the symptoms progress slowly and worsen over time. It can be deadly. In fact, COPD is the fourth-leading cause of death of Americans. According to the Centers for Disease Control, in the year 2000, 120,000 men and women in the United States died of COPD.

But America has no monopoly on COPD deaths. Worldwide, almost three million deaths are attributed to COPD each year in countries as diverse as Thailand, Japan, China, Egypt, Brazil, Croatia, France, Great Britain, and the Netherlands. According to researcher Susan Ward of the Centre for Exercise Science and Medicine at the University of Glasgow in Scotland, it is predicted that by the year 2020, chronic obstructive pulmonary disease will be the third-leading cause of death worldwide. Even today, COPD is second only to heart disease as a cause of disability in adults younger than sixty-five years of age.

COPD affects more men than women, although in the last ten years, the rates of women diagnosed with COPD have increased by 30 percent. That's due to the increased incidence of smoking among women over the last half of the twentieth century and because smoking is the number one cause of COPD.

SELF-EDUCATION IS IMPORTANT

It's important to understand what actually happens to your lungs (and you) when you have emphysema and chronic bronchitis, as well as how to recognize symptoms when they appear so you can receive treatment as soon as possible. This is vital because by the time you begin to experience symptoms, irreversible lung damage has already occurred. But although COPD cannot be cured, it can be treated, and when you stop smoking, you can slow the progression of the disease.

Why do you need to know all this? Because the more informed you and family members are about COPD, the more quickly you can receive a diagnosis, begin treatment, and learn how to live as fully as possible with your disease as it progresses. You will become the most important member of your health care team. Education makes the difference between being able to enjoy life, even with the burdens inflicted by COPD, by making the necessary modifications, or withdrawing from the world and allowing the disease to dictate your existence.

Although a book such as this can never substitute for the information you should receive from your physician and your rehabilitation program, it may answer many of your questions in more detail. As managed care restrictions limit the amount of time a physician can spend with each patient (about eighteen minutes, according to a Rutgers University study), you need to educate yourself and your family as completely as possible about your disease. Then you'll be more prepared to ask your health care provider specific questions when you meet.

THE SIGNS AND SYMPTOMS OF COPD

The signs and symptoms of COPD gradually sneak up on you, but the most common symptom is shortness of breath accompanied by coughing and/or wheezing and an abundance of sputum (also called phlegm), caused by chronic bronchial irritation.

■ Chronic Bronchitis

Although many people suffer from bronchitis (an inflammation of the bronchi), especially when they have an upper respiratory infection, it isn't considered to be a chronic condition unless the symptoms—a productive cough that brings up sputum—occur for three straight months for two consecutive years. You don't necessarily need to have trouble breathing; you can have nonobstructive chronic bronchitis, which just involves a cough without any shortness of breath.

Chronic bronchitis often develops in people over age forty who are or were moderate to heavy smokers. It occurs when the airways in your lungs, irritated for years by cigarette smoke, narrow from scarring and become clogged with excessive mucus that you try to bring up by coughing. This combination makes it difficult for air to pass through.

■ Emphysema

Emphysema is usually diagnosed in smokers or ex-smokers (usually fifty to seventy-five years of age). They suffer from fatigue and shortness of breath, which at first is noticeable only on heavy exercise, but as the disease progresses, the breathlessness increases until it occurs even on the lightest of activity. This triggers depression and the inclination to do less and less in order to prevent being breathless, but ironically, this action (or more accurately, the lack of it) causes the individual to become physically less conditioned and more fatigued.

In emphysema, the alveoli, the air sacs deep within the lungs, become damaged and then rupture and are destroyed. This makes large holes in the lungs that trap air, making it difficult for the lungs to perform the exchange of oxygen and carbon dioxide. Having lost their elasticity, the air sacs can no longer expel carbon dioxide during expiration, so breathing becomes more labored. The stagnant air in the alveoli can't supply adequate oxygen to the capillaries to service the rest of the body. It also creates a fertile field in which bacteria can grow. At the same time, carbon dioxide levels increase in the blood, causing fatigue, headaches, and a sense of lethargy.

The most common cause of emphysema is smoking, although other factors, such as air pollution, cooking in nonventilated areas, and a genetic component, may contribute to it as well.

■ Alpha-1-antitrypsin Deficiency

This is a rare genetic form of emphysema caused by a deficiency of the enzyme alpha-1-antitrypsin (AAT), a substance needed to protect the lungs' elastic fibers. AAT is produced by the liver and is a "lung protector." People suffering from this deficiency are predisposed to developing a rapid form of emphysema, often in their forties. If individuals with this condition are smokers, their symptoms may begin even earlier.

According to the American Lung Association, AAT is responsible for about 5 percent of the emphysema in the United States. An estimated 50,000 to 100,000 Americans, primarily of northern European descent, have AAT deficiency.

■ Asthma

Asthma is also a disease of the lungs, one that affects more than 15 million Americans and more than 100 million people worldwide. Fortunately, it is reversible. Unfortunately, however, asthma is on the increase and sometimes can be fatal. Asthma kills about five thousand Americans each year.

When specific triggers, which differ from person to person, affect the bronchial tubes, the lining of these airways swells, produces more mucus, and makes it difficult to breathe. People with asthma may cough, trying to force the mucus out, and wheeze as they then try to suck air in through their swollen airways.

There are a number of triggers for asthma, ranging from dust, animal dander, pollens, and mold to cold air, tobacco smoke, acid reflux (when stomach acid backs up into the esophagus in a condition known as gastroesophageal reflux disease or GERD), smog, and strong odors such as perfume or cleaning products. For some individuals, exercise, respiratory infections, laughing, or even eating triggers their asthma.

Unlike emphysema and chronic bronchitis, however, asthma attacks tend to be episodic, which means they come and go. Also differing from emphysema and chronic bronchitis, asthma symptoms can be controlled with proper and prompt medication.

■ Breathlessness

Breathlessness comes on gradually with the diseases of COPD. At first, you may notice only being out of breath while performing strenuous activity, such as when you're climbing stairs, playing tennis, running to catch a bus, or chasing after kids or grandkids. But eventually, the breathlessness occurs as you're making the bed, walking, holding up your arms as you read your newspaper, hitting a golf ball, shaving, putting away dishes, or brushing your hair. Simple activities of daily life become exhausting. It's frustrating and depressing, which in themselves are fatiguing factors. That's the point at which many people tend to reduce their activities and withdraw from social events. Unfortunately, it also is often the point at which they finally seek medical treatment.

■ Coughing

Coughing is another major symptom of COPD. It's partly caused by the fact that the normal mucus that lines the airways, which have become narrowed, is increased and thickened. Patients are urged to try to cough the mucus (also known as "phlegm," "spit," or "gunk") up as much as possible, as leaving it can make individuals more susceptible to infection as well as clogging their airways. Staying well hydrated by drinking eight eight-ounce glasses of water daily can help thin out the mucus and make it easier to cough up.

In a study funded by the pharmaceutical company Glaxo-SmithKline, 76 percent of patients with COPD interviewed said they coughed at least a few days a week while 53 percent acknowledged that they coughed every day. Twenty-three percent said they were awakened every night due to coughing, wheezing, or shortness of breath.

The Lung Association of Canada offers these suggestions for controlled coughing:

1. Take a slow, deep breath and hold it for two seconds.
2. Cough twice, with your mouth slightly open. The first cough should loosen mucus and the second cough should propel it out of the lungs.

3. Pause for a few seconds. Relax. Can be repeated if needed, but mucus plug should have been expelled.
4. Sniff gently. Do not take in a deep breath, as this may cause you to cough again and drive the mucus back into the lungs.
5. Rest.

■ Warning Signs That Things Are Getting Worse

In addition to knowing the signs and symptoms of COPD, it is important to know when your condition has worsened and you need to get immediate medical attention. Ask yourself these questions. If the answer to any question is yes, call your physician right away or go to the emergency department of your nearest hospital.

- Am I more breathless than usual, even when doing light activity?
- Am I more fatigued, even to the point of not wanting to get up or eat?
- Has the sputum I'm coughing up changed in color, such as now green, yellow, or brown?
- Is there an unusual increase or decrease in the amount of sputum?
- Has the consistency of the sputum become thicker or stickier?
- Is there blood in the sputum?
- Am I coughing more than previously?
- When I inhale and exhale, does it make a wheezing sound?
- Am I running a fever? (Don't guess; use a thermometer.)

- Do I have trouble getting to sleep and remaining asleep?
- Do I have swelling in my ankles or legs?
- Do I pant in order to catch my breath?
- Do my lips and fingertips have a bluish cast?
- Do I feel anxious, as though I can't get enough air?
- Do I have chest pain?

HOW LUNGS FUNCTION NORMALLY

Think of your lungs as a magnificent recycling machine bringing in oxygen that enters the bloodstream to nourish the body's tissues when you inhale and expelling the waste product of carbon dioxide when you exhale. Normally, a healthy person processes (breathes in and out) 5,000 gallons (18,940 liters) of air every day.

Although you have two lungs, they don't look the same, other than the color. Healthy lungs appear pink and spongy. Your right lung has three lobes or sections while your left lung has only two sections in order to make room for your heart. The bottoms of both lungs rest on your diaphragm, a thick, flat muscle that separates your lung area from your abdominal organs. The lungs themselves have no muscles; they are moved by the diaphragm and your chest muscles. When you breathe in, the diaphragm flattens and your chest muscles draw the ribs outward. This causes a bellowslike action that pulls air into the lungs and pushes to help expel it.

■ Air in, Air Out

When you breathe (either through your mouth or nose), you draw in air, and it flows down your windpipe or *trachea*. The windpipe lies alongside the esophagus, the tube carrying food from your mouth to your stomach. (When food "goes down the wrong way," that means some of it may have gone into the windpipe by mistake.)

The windpipe is about 4½ inches (11.4 centimeters) long with a diameter of about 1 inch (2.5 centimeters). It is held permanently open by a series of about twenty C-shaped rings of cartilage, a thick, fibrous connective tissue that normally allows easy passage of air. This main tube, the windpipe or trachea, branches into two smaller tubes. Think of it as a main river flowing into two tributaries, carrying not water but oxygen-rich air. Each of these two tributaries is called a *bronchus*, with one leading to the left lung and the other to the right. Both then divide into smaller airways called *bronchi*. It may help to think of these smaller structures as streams branching off from the tributary, dividing and then subdividing, getting smaller with each divide. Minuscule muscles surround these airways, automatically relaxing or contracting as the air passes through, much like a dam on a river controls the flow of water. All the time, air rich in oxygen is flowing through these tiny passages.

These bronchi keep getting smaller and smaller, dividing into fifteen to twenty-five minute airways called *bronchioles* and even smaller *alveolar ducts*. These airways end in clusters of grapelike bubbles or sacs called *alveoli*. Each lung has approximately 300 million of these little sacs. It is often said that if all the alveoli in both lungs were spread flat, they would cover an area about the size of a regulation tennis court. The alveoli are filled with microscopic blood vessels called *capillaries*, and this is where the action is. Oxygen floating in air brought into the lungs passes through the ultra-thin membrane making up the walls of the

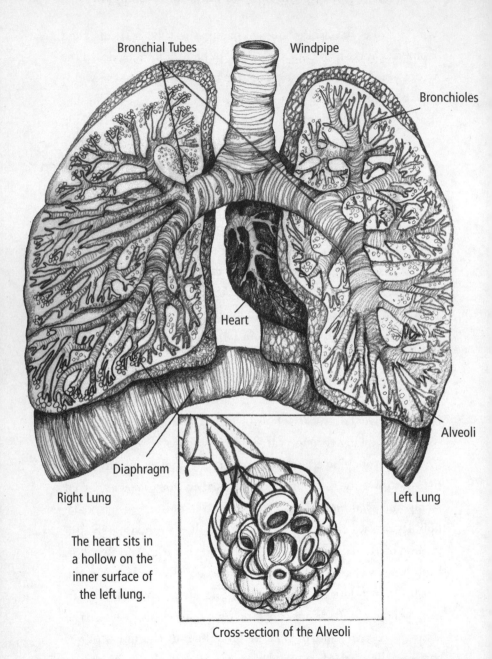

Bronchial Tubes   Windpipe

Bronchioles

Heart

Alveoli

Diaphragm

Right Lung

Left Lung

The heart sits in
a hollow on the
inner surface of
the left lung.

Cross-section of the Alveoli

Illustration © Kathy Taylor Zimmerman

alveoli and is absorbed into the capillaries and then into the bloodstream, to be pumped by the left side of the heart where it is disbursed as needed throughout the body. The waste product, carbon dioxide, is released from the capillaries into the alveoli and breathed out during expiration. This process is called *respiration* or *exhalation*.

■ Lungs Play "Cleanup"

The lungs have a second function besides their job of bringing in oxygen and expelling carbon dioxide. When you inhale through your nose, dust particles, pollutants, and bacteria in the air are filtered out by tiny hairs in the nose called *cilia* or are trapped by the sticky layer of mucus that lines the nasal passages.

The lungs have a filtering system for material that gets past the nose and nasal passages. The airways also are covered with a slippery substance that is actually a group of cells called *epithelial* cells. These cells act as a padding to protect the airways. Other cells produce mucus to catch irritants that slip by the primary line of defense in the nose. Some cells in the airways, like those in the nasal passages, also have tiny hairs called *cilia*, which act in unison like the oarsmen you see in a racing shell, directed by an unseen coxswain as they push the mucus with its captured impurities away from the lungs and upward to the throat (to be coughed out or swallowed), then fall back to push in rhythm again.

Fortunately, breathing is automatic, and when things are going well, you don't think about it. But when problems exist, as they do with asthma, chronic bronchitis, emphysema, and COPD, you can no longer take breathing for granted. As the American

Lung Association says in its motto, "If You Can't Breathe, Nothing Else Matters."

WHAT CAUSES COPD?

▪ Smoking Is the Most Important Risk Factor for COPD

Although a number of factors contribute to COPD, the number one risk factor is smoking, a dreadful addiction still actively promoted by subtle advertising, social and peer pressure, and the media. It's estimated that 80 to 90 percent of people diagnosed with COPD have had considerable exposure to tobacco smoke (either by smoking at least twenty cigarettes a day for twenty or more years or by inhaling secondhand smoke for many years).

This means that COPD is largely preventable and could be downgraded to a minor health problem if people didn't smoke. Instead, COPD is on the increase despite the fact that more people (at least in the United States) are giving up the smoking habit. Unfortunately, because it takes twenty or more years for smoking to affect the lungs to the point that it causes symptoms, most people are unaware of the damage that's occurring in their body until it's too late. And don't think that switching to a pipe or cigar will change that statistic. According to pulmonologist Lee Kirkman, "If you've been a former cigarette smoker and change to a pipe or cigar, you will still inhale."

It really is a gamble—a dangerous one—because not everyone who takes up smoking gets COPD. Experts say that if you're a smoker, you have between a one-in-four and one-in-six chance of getting COPD. Researchers still aren't sure what predisposes some smokers to COPD and others to escape this devastating disease. Nevertheless, the fact remains that 80 to 90 percent of patients with COPD were or are smokers.

What Smoking Does to the Lungs

Remember the description of the respiratory system? Microscopic hairs called cilia line the bronchial tubes. Their purpose is to sweep out germs and other irritants, like tobacco smoke, that find their way into the bronchi. But tobacco smoke paralyzes these hairs, rendering them useless. The germs and irritants remain in the bronchial tubes, inflaming the delicate membranes and eventually clogging them, which also makes them more prone to infections.

■ Environmental Causes

Although smoking is the primary cause of COPD, it isn't the only one. People living and working in polluted areas—both indoors and out-of-doors—are more susceptible to COPD. According to the American Lung Association's State of the Air 2002 report, "more than 142 million Americans—75 percent of the nation's population living in counties with ozone monitors—are breathing unhealthy amounts of ozone air pollution (smog)."

Certain professions, such as those involved with chemical fumes, fabric, fiberglass, or other microscopic fibers, extreme dampness, or dust, also put their workers at a higher risk for developing COPD. Even hobbies such as painting, woodworking, or those requiring the use of aerosol sprays can make you more susceptible to developing COPD.

■ **Respiratory Infections**

Frequent respiratory infections, especially in childhood, can cause injury to the delicate membranes of the lungs. That's why doctors urge their patients to get an annual flu shot as well as a vaccination against pneumonia, which protects for five to seven years (not for a lifetime as originally thought). According to researchers, an annual flu vaccination reduces serious illness and mortality in COPD by about half.

Two of the most common contributory causes of respiratory infection are at the ends of your arms: your hands. Wash your hands frequently, especially after using the toilet, changing a diaper, visiting a hospital or nursing home, shaking hands at social gatherings, or just being outdoors. Also wash your hands before eating or preparing food. Experts suggest you sing "Happy Birthday" (preferably to yourself!) as you wash your hands with warm water and soap to be sure you've washed long enough. Be sure to scrub under your fingernails, too.

Stay away from crowds or people who have respiratory infections. You may be extremely susceptible, especially if you're fatigued or your immune system is otherwise lowered.

■ **Genetic Predisposition**

As mentioned above, there is one rare cause of COPD that is genetic, alpha-1-antitrypsin deficiency. Those with this insufficiency of the protein antitrypsin are more prone to developing COPD and at an earlier age than those who develop it from smoking or any of the other external causes.

■ **Family Clustering**

There does seem to be what researchers call "family clusters" as a contributing cause of COPD. This means that it tends to run in families. If your parents or grandparents had emphysema or chronic bronchitis, you may be more prone to it as well. Whether the clustering effect is due to genetic defects or environmental or socioeconomic influences, or a combination of some or all of these factors, has as yet not been determined.

MYTHS ABOUT COPD

Despite the fact that chronic obstructive pulmonary disease is the fourth largest cause of death in the United States and afflicts more people than diabetes, it is still often misdiagnosed by physicians and is totally unknown to many people. Those who have heard of COPD are sometimes confused by many myths surrounding this chronic and progressive disease.

Myth: Although smoking is the number one cause of chronic obstructive pulmonary disease, you are cured once you stop smoking.

TRUTH: Smoking *is* the number one cause of COPD. But although it's important to stop smoking, the damage to the lungs is permanent. Chronic obstructive pulmonary disease is progressive, meaning it gets worse, not better.

Myth: COPD is a man's disease.

TRUTH: COPD used to be considered a man's disease when more men smoked, but as women began smoking heavily during and after World War II, the number of women with COPD began to rise and now almost equals that of men. With young women now smoking in larger numbers than young men, the

incidence of COPD in the future may become higher among
the female population.

Myth: People with COPD should not exercise because it
makes them breathless.

TRUTH: Physician-approved exercise is vital for those with
COPD because it helps to maintain strength and conditions
muscles so they require less oxygen to function adequately. Exercise also makes a person with COPD feel better about his or her
body and improves the quality of life.

Myth: People with COPD are breathless only when they
exercise.

TRUTH: People with COPD often suffer from breathlessness
even when they have engaged in no strenuous physical activity.
They can have dyspnea (shortness of breath) while in bed, sitting and reading, or just eating or talking.

Myth: COPD is an old person's disease.

TRUTH: Although most COPD patients are fifty or older,
there is a genetic predisposition to a form of emphysema before
age fifty that then develops into COPD. Onset varies, with
those who smoke experiencing shortness of breath even in their
mid-thirties.

Myth: With proper medication, your COPD symptoms will
clear up.

TRUTH: Unfortunately, no current medication can reverse the
damage caused by COPD. It can, however, lessen some of the
symptoms of the disease.

Myth: COPD is contagious, so you should stay away from people who cough.

TRUTH: COPD is not a contagious disease. If you have it, however, you should stay away from people who have respiratory infections because you are more susceptible to catching them.

Myth: COPD is another name for asthma.

TRUTH: COPD is the name given to a combination of disorders including chronic bronchitis, emphysema, and, sometimes, asthma. However, asthma can be controlled by medications and normally is not progressive, whereas COPD is a chronic and progressive disease that destroys the effectiveness of the lungs.

2

How COPD Is Diagnosed

How do you know if you have COPD and when should you see a doctor? These are probably two of the most important questions because most people don't seek medical attention soon enough, until permanent lung damage has already occurred. It's important to know and recognize the early signs of COPD so treatment can begin and in order to slow the progression of the disease.

WHEN TO SEE A DOCTOR

If you're a smoker, you may be so used to waking up with a hacking cough that you don't think much about it, even though you're coughing up thick yellow or green sputum. It's easy to be in denial and think it's just a "smoker's cough" or a "simple" chest cold. But if you've been coughing for more than a couple of weeks or find that you're feeling short of breath when you walk or climb stairs, lift grocery bags or laundry baskets, or just feel tired all the time, please see your doctor. You may have COPD, and although the damage to your lungs is permanent and cannot be reversed, prompt and effective treatment can slow the progress of the disease.

THE DOCTOR-PATIENT RELATIONSHIP

Selecting a doctor when you have a chronic condition like COPD is far different from looking for one who can treat your sore throat or rash. You're both in it for the long haul, so you have a number of issues to consider. In addition to choosing someone who is knowledgeable about your disease and its treatment, it's important to find a physician with whom you feel comfortable, as you'll be spending a great deal of time together.

Obviously, some factors may act as a barrier to your making a satisfying selection. You may live in a small town without many physicians to choose from. Your insurance plan may also limit your options by giving you coverage with only one or two physicians. If you or your spouse is employed, your company may change insurance companies and you'll find yourself unable to continue with the doctor with whom you have developed a relationship. You find yourself back at square one, trying to find the right doctor for you. And that "for you" is an important qualifier to remember because the physician your friend raves about may not be the right one for you.

HOW TO FIND A QUALIFIED PHYSICIAN

- Ask a physician you trust for a list of physicians she would recommend and use herself, if it were needed.

- Check with your local American Lung Association for a list of qualified physicians in your area.
- Contact an area hospital.
- If you live near a medical school, ask for names of physicians who deal with lung disorders.
- Call the Lung Line of the National Jewish Medical Research Center in Denver. It is a well-respected and well-known center for research and treatment of lung diseases. Their Lung Line is open Monday through Friday from 8 A.M. to 5 P.M. mountain time. If you live outside Colorado, call 800-222-LUNG. If you're calling from Colorado, call 303-398-1477.

MEET THE DOCTORS

▪ Primary Care Physician

Probably the first physician you'll see when you become aware of your symptoms is your regular doctor, the person you go to when something hurts or you just "don't feel well." He or she is likely an internist, family care physician, or general practitioner (GP). All of these have been trained in primary care medicine, so-called because they see patients first. They diagnose and treat you from head to toe, from the weird rash that won't go away, to inflamed tonsils, to the stubbed toe you think may be broken. Just as important, they can all recognize situations that require sending you to a specialist.

Although internists, family doctors, and general practitioners all have had training in treating pulmonary (lung) diseases, they do not specialize in this area. For that, you need to see a pulmonologist.

■ Pulmonologist

If their insurance plan permits, many people bypass an internist and head right for a pulmonologist when they begin to have problems breathing. Pulmonologists are physicians who first spend three years specializing in internal medicine. They then train for two additional years with a fellowship in pulmonary medicine at an accredited institution. In addition, these physicians must take and pass national examinations to become "board certified."

WHY THE DOCTOR-PATIENT RELATIONSHIP IS SO IMPORTANT

The relationship between you and your physician is of utmost importance because it can affect the quality of your treatment. As with all relationships—personal and business—there has to be mutual trust. You need to feel comfortable giving honest answers to questions about how you're following (or not) medical instructions, alcohol and illegal drug use, smoking, and exercise. As you will often be sharing your deepest emotions, fears, and details of your personal life, you need to know that the doctor will keep your confidences, take your concerns seriously, and really listen to what you have to say.

TRUE COMMUNICATION REQUIRES LISTENING AS WELL AS TALKING

Although you may have been talking since you were about fourteen months old, you may not have learned how to communicate effectively, and that's a very important skill, especially when you have a chronic illness such as COPD. Even if you are hesitant to express yourself or share your feelings, this is the time to begin. As Ralph Waldo Emerson wrote, "It's a luxury to be understood."

When you have COPD, it's more than a luxury to be understood, it's a necessity. Your life may depend on how good a team you and your physician become. We talk to people every day, but often it isn't very effective. Others don't understand our messages while we assume that they have; we aren't really listening to their response because we're thinking of what we're going to answer back; and we're including a subtext that really isn't very well explained or are using body language that negates our message. Welcome to the modern-day Tower of Babel.

Also, remember that our vocabulary sometimes limits meanings. "I'm fine" can mean, "I feel crummy, but I'm dealing with it okay" or "I'm feeling pretty good," or, depending on how it is expressed, "Stop asking me." Unless your doctor is also a mind reader, he or she will be in the dark or, worse, take your words at their face value.

In addition, every profession has its own jargon and acronyms that those in the field speak fluently but that leave most outsiders confused. To communicate effectively with your physician and other health care officials, you're going to have to take a crash course in Medical Jargon 101.

Although the "Words to Know" section in the back of this book lists many terms that you'll need to know as you cope with COPD, either as a patient or a caregiver, there are others that you'll hear from your physician or other health care providers. Don't guess at their meaning; ask for a definition. Then write the word down in your notebook along with the definition and, if necessary, how the word is pronounced.

Learn the names, description, and purpose of the medications you take so you can discuss them by name, rather than "the little white pill I take in the morning." Doctors are human. When they see you making the effort to become educated in your disease and trying to speak their language, they usually bend over backward to be helpful and give you the attention you deserve when you need to speak to them. They know that you are aware of their time constraints, have concise questions, and are focused on their responses. It's hard for even the busiest physician not to appreciate your consideration and to return it in kind.

Only you can know your symptoms from your personal perspective. That's what makes everyone a unique individual with COPD, rather than "a COPD case." While the doctor should be an expert in COPD and have seen hundreds of patients with the disease, he or she doesn't know your fears, how the condition is personally affecting you, your life, and your relationships. There needs to be true communication going on—with you talking, the doctor listening and then reflecting back to you what has been heard so there's no "assuming" or misunderstanding. When the doctor gives you options, it's important for you to listen and give feedback as well, so he or she doesn't assume that you understand (when you don't) or will comply (when you won't).

This two-way exchange with both listening and talking, and the sharing of ideas, feelings, concerns, and advice is so important because you don't exist in a vacuum. You may have family and other responsibilities that are affected by treatment choices. Unless the doctor understands what's going on in your life, he or she may not know why you are questioning specific aspects of your treatment. Research has shown that medical treatments are more successful when doctors consider a patient's emotions and life circumstances in addition to his or her disease.

Effective communication is honest communication. The doctor doesn't have to waste time and energy wondering what your *real* message is. When you say, "I'm fine," your physician will understand that you're having a good day. If you're not and you answer, "I had a slight setback, and it scares me," the medical professional will know your status and be available to offer support, comfort and, often, information that may be helpful. He or she won't have to wonder whether to take you at your word or if there's a subtext that he or she just isn't getting.

OPEN COMMUNICATION CAN BE SCARY

It's a little frightening to open up if you aren't used to it, to share your thoughts and feelings with someone who's almost a total stranger, wears a white coat, and occasionally uses terms that make it sound as though he or she is speaking in tongues. But once you've tried to express your innermost thoughts, it comes easier the next time.

I know this to be true, personally, because I had always tried to be strong and not share my fears. But the night after my diagnosis with breast cancer, I remember lying in my husband's arms. "I'm scared," I confided in a small voice.

He didn't try to talk me out of my feelings or recite statistics on the odds of total recovery from breast cancer. Instead, he held me closely and said, "You'd be foolish if you weren't." He acknowledged my feelings, was nonjudgmental, and remained supportive and available as I considered my options.

This "feeling feedback" is important because it validates your feelings and allows the physician to acknowledge how you feel as a part of the communication process. When we recognize and acknowledge another's feelings, we give them form and substance. Instead of floating around like vapor in the atmosphere, our feelings become tangible and we can deal with them.

Physicians often struggle to maintain effective communication with their patients. Your physician may have "inherited" faulty communication skills from his or her family, where feelings were hidden behind a No Trespassing sign. And, although medical schools spend a great deal of time instructing their students how to take a medical history, too little attention is given to perfecting effective communication skills including speaking *and* listening.

When you meet with your doctor, your tone may be light and your gestures dismissive of your underlying concerns. The doctor's mind may wander while listening to what you're saying, causing him or her to miss your vocal or body language cues. There may be noises—conversation right outside of the examination room, honking horns outside the window, phones ringing, or computer printers clanking—disrupting your train of thought or that of your physician. Problems such as these can garble both the transmission and the receiving of messages, often with disturbing results.

That's when you need to speak up and ask the doctor to close the door, or pause while the jet is flying overhead until you can be heard again. We really aren't isolated islands—doctor and patient. It's just that we need to build bridges to help us reach out to each other.

COMPLIANCE IS IMPORTANT

Compliance comes from a Latin word meaning "to complete." It doesn't mean blindly following whatever orders the doctor gives you, however. It means that after discussing your options, side effects of the treatment plan, and long-range goals, you agree to comply with or follow through on the prescribed course of action. You are more likely to comply with the doctor's suggestions if you feel he or she considers you an important part of your health team.

Compliance is especially important for you because in treating COPD patients, medication is often prescribed in combination and over a period of many years. Yet perhaps as many as half of patients on long-term drug therapy don't take all their medication. In addition, some patients use more than the required dosage of some medications when their symptoms worsen, figuring that "more is better."

Compliance that comes after effective two-way communication between doctor and patient takes time. Unfortunately, studies published in *The New England Journal of Medicine* reveal that the average visit lasts just eighteen minutes (visits to female physicians are about one minute longer on average than those to male doctors). That's less time than a television sitcom, yet during that time the doctor is expected to gain information on your condition and how you're reacting to the various medications; discuss ways you can handle activities of daily living in order to live as normal a life as possible; answer your questions; explain new treatment plans; educate you about your disease; encourage you to exercise, eat a balanced diet, and stop smoking; while also offering reassurance and support. It's no easy task.

This two-way transfer of information *can* take place. It just takes time and effort on both your parts, as well as the physician's staff. As the receptionist and nurses get to know you, they must learn that when you call with a problem, it's not trivial. It may be an issue familiar to them, but it's new to you. On the other hand, you must also do your part by understanding before leaving the doctor's office all of his or her instructions including how and when to take all of your medications, so you don't have to call unless it really is important.

Many excellent physicians have no idea what goes on in their front office, either with their receptionist or office staff. One doctor told me, "I'm so busy seeing patients, I have no time to train my staff. I never have staff meetings!" Yet an efficient and effective front office can answer many of your questions, reduce your stress, and be meaningful partners to the physician they serve. If you have a problem with the doctor's staff, let him or her know.

ARE YOU AND YOUR DOCTOR A GOOD "FIT"?

Doctors, like the rest of us, have personality traits that have nothing to do with their professional skills. Unfortunately, because of the personal relationship that must develop between a physician and a patient with a chronic illness, your personalities need to mesh. If you want to know everything that's happening to you, and your doctor is of the don't-you-worry-your-pretty-little-head school, it's not going to be an effective relationship. Nor will it be if your doctor continually goes into scientific explanations and obscure studies while your eyes glaze over and you wonder when he'll get to "just the facts, ma'am."

It's your job to be up front with your physician from the start about just how much information you want to hear. What may seem an insignificant issue to your doctor may loom very large in your mind. As author Anaïs Nin wrote, "We don't see things as they are, we see things as we are." Try to find a physician who understands the difference.

Ask yourself these questions when assessing your physician and the office staff:

- When I call for an appointment, does the receptionist make me feel as though I'm intruding on the doctor's time?
- When I keep my appointment and am in the reception area, am I seen in a timely manner (within the hour) or am I kept waiting for hours without any comment from the staff as to the cause of the delay?
- Do I feel comfortable answering the doctor's questions about my personal life?
- Is the exam room private and quiet, or does noise or nurses popping in and out disturb us?
- Does my doctor keep up to date on new medications and treatments for COPD?
- Does my doctor take time to answer my list of questions, or is he a door hugger, inching toward the door even as I speak?
- Does my doctor explain information concerning my condition, tests, medications, and treatment in a way that I understand?
- If I don't understand, will my doctor take the time to explain in a way that helps me to understand, or at least refer me to a staff member who can do so?

- Does my doctor treat me as a partner in my treatment program, respecting my opinions concerning my care even if he or she doesn't agree with me?
- Does my doctor change the topic or seem uncomfortable when I express emotional, sexual, or psychological concerns arising from my condition?
- Has my doctor explained his or her philosophy about the treatment of COPD, pain control, and what to do in an emergency?
- Am I confident that my doctor will be available for me in an emergency?
- If my doctor is a sole practitioner, have I been told who will see me in an emergency if he or she is not available?
- Do I trust my doctor's judgment enough to comply with our agreed upon treatment program?

YOU HAVE RESPONSIBILITIES, TOO

Just as communication between doctor and patient must be a two-way exchange, you as a patient have responsibilities just as your physician has. These are your responsibilities:

- Give up smoking if you still do. Tell your doctor if you are having difficulty. He or she can suggest ways to help you kick the habit. (See Chapter 3 for ways to help you stop smoking.)
- Answer your doctor's questions honestly and to your best ability. And if you are sneaking cigarettes, admit it. Lying, especially about alcohol or drug usage, over-the-counter medications, or herbal remedies you are taking

may interfere with some of the medications being pre-scribed for you and could even have harmful results.

- Let your doctor know how much information you are ready to receive. Some people want an overview of their illness that focuses on just where they are at the present, while others want to know what may be in store for them down the road.
- Learn as much as you can about your disease by reading books (see "Suggested Reading" at the back of this book), joining a support group, or asking your physician specific questions about issues that concern you.
- Check sites relating to COPD on the Internet, but realize that not all of the information you find there is accurate. Stick to the sites sponsored by national organizations such as the American Lung Association, National Jewish Medical and Research Center, National Lung Health Education tion Program (NLHEP), the National Emphysema/COPD Association, or those of major hospitals.
- Follow your doctor's treatment plan, once all your questions have been answered to your satisfaction. That means using the medications exactly as prescribed (on an empty stomach or with meals, completing the prescription rather than stopping when you feel better, and so on), and following your exercise and diet plans as specified. If you can't afford all your medications, tell your doctor. Physicians often have samples that they can give to their patients when necessary.
- Tell your doctor if you don't understand something and ask him or her to restate it in a different way, or to give you reading material, a video, etc.

- Call your doctor if there are any changes in your condition, including a change in the color or amount of sputum, more difficulty with breathing, fever, cough, or more fatigue than usual.
- Respect the physician's time by calling only when necessary and asking to speak to the nurse if she can answer a question for you.
- Cancel an appointment (and reschedule it) if you are unable to keep it, rather than just not showing up.
- Make friends with the office staff. They usually have a lot of information. And they are the people who decide whether—or not—to disrupt the schedule with your emergency appointment.

PREPARE FOR YOUR OFFICE VISIT

In addition to seeing the doctor when symptoms change, you'll have regular appointments scheduled to measure your airflow and volume, check on how things are going for you in your day-to-day activities, and what medications may need to be changed or dosages altered. Plan ahead for these routine visits. You can make them more pleasant and effective in a number of ways.

- Bring something to read, as most of the magazines in the office are probably very out of date. If needlepointing or knitting doesn't tire you too much, bring it along to help the time pass more quickly.
- Be on time for your appointment. If one person arrives ten minutes late, it affects everyone else the doctor will see that day. Multiply that by a few patients coming in

late, and you realize why you may have to wait a while in the reception area (what they used to call the "waiting room").

- Bring a list of questions that you and other family members have about your medications and other treatments, exercise, planned trips, and so on. Don't trust those questions to memory.

- Take notes as the doctor gives you instructions. If it tires you, ask a friend or family member to come with you and take notes. You also can use a tape recorder, although technical equipment has been known to fail at times. Before you use the tape recorder, however, be sure your doctor understands why you want to tape the instructions and that he or she is comfortable with your doing so.

- If you don't understand the doctor's instructions, speak up and ask him or her to repeat them to you.

- If you're getting new medications, always ask about potential side effects if the doctor forgets to tell you. It's new to you, even though he or she has prescribed it hundreds of times. Remember, however, that few people get all or even some of the side effects. You may not have any, but it saves a phone call and needless worry if you do.

- If you're having trouble coping with your sense of isolation due to your COPD or your frustration at having to abandon some of the activities you once enjoyed—including sex—tell your doctor. It's nothing to be embarrassed about or ashamed of. Sometimes it helps just to have someone other than family listen to you.

Next to the love and support of your family and friends, the most important relationship you will develop over the years is with your physician. Select one wisely and be willing to give of yourself, be honest, communicate openly, and listen. It will help you deal with your disease more effectively and make life more pleasant because you know you have someone you can learn from and lean on when necessary.

THE PATIENT HISTORY

When you first see your doctor, he or she will take a medical history. This consists of an interview during which the physician (or physician's assistant) gathers information about you. He or she will ask you to describe your symptoms and tell when they first appeared, your smoking habits, your use of alcohol and other drugs (legal and illegal), your use of over-the-counter medications and herbal remedies, your occupation (do you work with paints, chemicals, diesel fumes, dust, aerosols, asbestos, grains, etc.), and whether your parents had emphysema, chronic bronchitis, or asthma, and if so, at what age. This last question is important because there seems to be a genetic propensity for COPD, especially if one or both of your parents were diagnosed with emphysema at an early age.

If the doctor asks you what your "chief complaint" is, don't think that means you're considered a complainer. It's medical jargon for, "What is the main reason you came for medical care?" The doctor also may ask if your cough is a "productive" one. This means, "Are you bringing up sputum?" If your answer is yes, be prepared to describe how much (a teaspoon, tablespoon, or half a cup); odor, if any; its consistency (thick or thin); and its color (clear, yellow, brown, or green). Be sure to answer these and other questions honestly and as accurately as you can.

Taking an accurate medical history is so important that medical school and nursing students all take specific courses in this subject. A carefully conducted medical history can help the doctor learn not only what your symptoms are but also how and when they appeared and to what extent they affect your daily activities.

THE PHYSICAL EXAMINATION

Then the physician will conduct a physical examination that includes, but is not limited to:

- checking your vital signs, which includes temperature, pulse rate, blood pressure, and respirations (breathing pattern).
- tapping your back (called *percussing*) to hear the sound of air density.
- listening to your heart and lungs with a stethoscope in order to detect abnormal sounds. To create agreement and conformity in discussing responses among physicians, the American Thoracic Society and the American College of Chest Physicians have categorized these sounds as *crackles* for discontinuous sounds and *wheezes* for the high-pitched whistling sounds.
- having you breathe in and out to see if you rely on neck muscles to help your weakened respiratory muscles move air. If this is the case, you may also have a barrel-shaped chest.

- checking your ankles and legs for swelling (called *peripheral edema*), which might signify fluid retention, a possible sign of heart complications.
- looking at your fingernails to see if they have a bluish tint (a condition called *cyanosis*), which could point to a lack of oxygen in your blood or clubbing, in which the diameter of the base of the fingernail is flattened and broader than the finger itself, and the nail itself is abnormally curved. It's a physical sign associated with certain chronic lung conditions.
- observing your skin tone to see if there is a bluish cast, which also might signify lack of sufficient oxygen in your blood.

DIAGNOSTIC TESTS

In addition to the physical examination, the doctor may suggest a number of tests in order to confirm the diagnosis of COPD. Most of these are noninvasive, which means not invading the body, unlike those done with blood work.

■ Pulmonary Function Test (PFT)

According to the NLHEP, the spirometry is the best single test for detecting early COPD. You will be asked to take a very deep breath and then blow out as hard and as fast as you can into the mouthpiece of a piece of equipment called a spirometer. The spirometer measures the amount of air that you can take into your lungs (called *volume*) and how fast you can blow air out (called *flow*). Sometimes you'll have the test done before and after you inhale medications in order to check your response to them. Speak up immediately if you feel dizzy or experience any chest pain, nausea, or wheezing.

The resulting amount of what you were able to exhale is known as the *forced vital capacity* or *FVC*. How much you were able to blow out in the first second is called the *forced expiratory volume in one second* or FEV_1. It's important that you know your results for these two numbers. Have your doctor explain what your numbers are and what they mean. Write your numbers down in your notebook and date them so you can compare the figures with future spirometry tests.

Spirometry is especially important for smokers because it can detect emphysema before your symptoms become obvious and debilitating.

■ Chest X-Ray

Your doctor will probably order front and side views of your chest in order to see your heart and lungs in order to ascertain what's causing your respiratory problem. You'll have to take a deep breath and hold it for a few seconds while the X ray is taken. Don't move or let out your breath until the technician tells you to. As a chest X-ray can be normal even with advanced stages of emphysema, the doctor probably will order other additional tests.

■ Electrocardiogram

This test is also called an EKG. Although it isn't too helpful in evaluating the extent of your COPD, it can detect abnormalities on the right side of the heart as it strains to pump blood back through the lungs to receive oxygen and dispel carbon dioxide. This may occur in very advanced stages of COPD.

▓ Computerized Tomography (CT) Scan

This noninvasive imaging test uses ultra-thin X-ray beams to take pictures that are then processed by a computer to allow your doctor to see your organs in a number of two-dimensional slices. A technician will position you on an X-ray table and may put a strap around your body to keep you in the proper position. Try not to move during the thirty to sixty minutes needed to complete the test, although you can breathe normally. CT scans are used to detect emphysema in more advanced stages.

▓ Sputum Analysis

By analyzing the cells in your sputum, your doctor can learn the cause of a lung problem, determining whether you have lung cancer, COPD, or an inflammatory process such as asthmatic bronchitis.

▓ Exercise Stress Test

This is also called a "stress test" or an "exercise test." It's usually conducted on a treadmill, so wear comfortable exercise clothes and athletic shoes. You'll be fitted with special equipment to measure your heart activity and breathing functions as you walk on the treadmill at varying speeds and levels. The purpose of this test is to determine your heart rate and oxygen usage during physical activity. You are constantly monitored during this test, so don't worry if you become too fatigued or too breathless to continue. The test can be easily halted at any time.

▓ Arterial Blood Gas Analysis (ABG)

This is an invasive test used to evaluate how effectively your lungs bring oxygen to the blood and remove carbon dioxide from it. However, it is more than a simple blood test—the blood sample must be taken from an artery in your wrist rather than from a vein.

Always ask the technician performing the test to first give you an injection of a local anesthetic, such as lidocaine, to deaden the area. Even with numbing medication, this procedure tends to be somewhat painful as arteries lie deeper in the body than veins, the artery in the wrist is close to a nerve, and arterial blood is under higher pressure. Nevertheless, the blood sample is usually taken from that artery inside the wrist because it is visible. It can, however, also be taken from your groin or the inside of your elbow.

Be sure to tell the physician or technician if you are on blood-thinning medication such as warfarin (coumadin) and report any other medications—prescription or over-the-counter or herbal remedies—as they may prevent your blood from clotting properly.

▪ Pulse Oximetry

This is a noninvasive test. It's a little clip like a clothespin that fits on the tip of your finger or on your earlobe. The oximeter measures the amount of oxygen in your blood and may be used to determine if you need supplemental oxygen when you exercise or sleep.

▪ Additional Blood Work

Another blood test checks for low alpha-1-antitrypsin levels, which would be suspected if you are under fifty years of age and a nonsmoker who displays signs of emphysema.

3

Treatments for COPD

Although there is no cure for COPD, there are a number of ways to treat the disease to make you more comfortable and to improve your quality of life. As Martina Navratilova, the Czech-American tennis champion, said, "Just go out there and do what you've got to do."

If you smoke, the most important thing to do is to stop. Additional treatments include medications that you ingest, inject, or inhale; pulmonary rehabilitation; supplemental oxygen; vaccinations; and surgery. Your individual treatment plan depends on many factors, including the course of your disease, other medical conditions you have, and the way your symptoms impact your activities of daily living.

According to the National Heart, Lung, and Blood Institute, the goal of any treatment plan is to help prevent and relieve your symptoms and to help you manage the effects of the disease and live a more active and enjoyable life. Together, you and your doctor can develop a complete respiratory care program that:

- improves lung function
- reduces hospitalizations
- prevents acute episodes
- minimizes disability
- prevents early death

YOU SHOULD SHARE YOUR DOCTOR'S PHILOSOPHY ABOUT TREATMENT

The key, as I stress over and over, is for you and your physician to work closely together. The doctor can't help you without your wholehearted involvement and complete cooperation. Your particular physician's philosophy is important, too. All physicians take the Hippocratic oath that says, "*Primum, non nocere,*" "First, do no harm." For some doctors, that means playing it conservatively and avoiding medications or combinations of medications and treatments that may bring on side effects that are more unpleasant for the patients than their original symptoms. Others believe in "full speed ahead," making available to their patients every weapon in their arsenal in order to slow the advancement of this progressive chronic disease. Most physicians are scattered somewhere along the continuum when it comes to their philosophies concerning treatment, but you should know and feel comfortable with whatever philosophy your physician holds. If you don't, seek out another doctor whose viewpoint you do share.

SMOKING: WHY YOU *MUST* STOP

Unless you've been trapped in space for the last ten years or been stranded on an ice floe in the Antarctic, you know that smoking is bad for you in many ways. From the economic aspect alone, smoking is an expensive habit. Just one pack a day costs about $1,000 a year, and that figure is rapidly escalating as many states are finding cigarettes an easy target on which to place high taxes, sometimes raising the price to as much as $7 per pack. And smokers find themselves targeted as well, as forty-six states forbid smoking in public places.

It probably comes as no surprise to you, but it bears repeating that smoking:

- increases the risk of cancer of the lung, mouth, larynx, and esophagus
- increases the risk of cancer of the bladder, stomach, kidney, pancreas, and, if you're a female, the cervix
- doubles your risk of heart disease, America's number one killer
- increases your risk of stroke, the number three cause of death in America
- increases the likelihood of pregnant women delivering prematurely and having babies of lower birth weight
- increases the risk of stroke, heart attack, and blood clots in women who use oral contraceptives
- increases the risk of developing—and dying from— stomach ulcers
- may cause errors in various diagnostic tests
- can cause deadly fires due to falling asleep while smoking in bed
- may affect the effectiveness of some of the medications you take, by either making them stronger or less effective than they should be. Some examples are as follows:

- Ulcer medicines such as Tagamet and Zantac
- Asthma medicines with theophylline such as Theo-Dur and Slo-Bid
- Anxiety medications such as Valium, Versed, and Librium
- Calcium channel blockers such as Procardia and Calan
- Nitrates used for angina/congestive heart failure such as Nitro-Dur and Nitrostat
- Migraine medications such as Migrex and Ergota-mine
- Diarrhea medications such as Kaopectate
- Over-the-counter antacids such as Mylanta, Tums, Maalox, and many others

If all of the above problems aren't frightening enough, smoking leads to chronic bronchitis and is the major cause of emphysema, a disease that slowly destroys your ability to breathe. The nicotine in the cigarettes prevents the cilia, the microscopic protective hairs that line your airways, from moving bacteria, dust, and other irritants out of the lungs. Instead, the bacteria and irritants nestle in the warm, moist areas of the lungs, causing infection that eventually triggers permanent damage to your bronchial tubes and the alveoli. The reaction to these irritative effects and the inflammatory response is that your lungs begin to secrete excess mucus that builds up in your airways and makes you cough.

Here is the bottom line, according to Paul Scanlon, M.D., a pulmonologist at the Mayo Clinic and a member of the recent Lung Health Study Research Group: "The only intervention that slows the progression of disease in COPD is smoking cessation."

■ Smoking Is an Addiction

Don't consider cigarette smoking to be just a "habit." It is far more than that. The nicotine found in cigarettes makes smoking an addiction because, according to the National Institute on Drug Abuse, nicotine use fulfills all the criteria of an addiction: compulsive drug-seeking and use, even in the face of negative health consequences; induces feelings of pleasure that serves as a reinforcer of its use; and creates typical withdrawal symptoms when not being used.

Cigarette smoking produces a rapid distribution of nicotine to the brain, with drug levels peaking within ten seconds of inhalation. Unfortunately, the acute effects of nicotine dissipate in a few minutes, causing the smoker to continue dosing frequently throughout the day to maintain the drug's pleasurable effects and prevent withdrawal. That's why cigarette smokers reach for a cigarette the first thing in the morning.

What people frequently don't realize is that the cigarette is a very efficient and highly engineered drug-delivery system. By inhaling, a smoker can get nicotine to the brain very rapidly with every puff. A typical smoker will take ten puffs on a cigarette during the five minutes that the cigarette is lit. Thus, a person who smokes about 1½ packs (30 cigarettes) daily, gets 300 "hits" of nicotine to the brain each day. These factors contribute considerably to nicotine's highly addictive nature.

University of Vermont professor John Hughes, past president of the Society for Research on Nicotine and Tobacco and an expert of nicotine dependence, says the scientific consensus is that "the core of the issue [over dependence] is the loss of control over use. The drug controls you—you don't control the drug."

Presently, tobacco companies are turning their attentions to capture the young adult market. Tragically, in twenty to thirty years, these populations will become the new crop of COPD patients as most patients with COPD have smoked at least twenty cigarettes per day for twenty or more years.

■ It Isn't Too Late to Stop Smoking

Your years of smoking have caught up with you and your lungs. You may feel, "What good will it do to stop? I've already got COPD, so how can smoking hurt me now?" It can. Although you can't reverse the damage already done to your lungs, you can slow the progress of the disease by preventing additional deterioration of the 300 million clusters of alveoli, that vital area deep in your lungs where life-generating oxygen is transferred into the bloodstream and carbon dioxide is expelled.

When you stop smoking, you'll have less phlegm to cough up, fewer incidents of respiratory infections, and less wheezing. You'll have less breathlessness, too. Even if you've tried to stop smoking before, you must try again. It can take anywhere from four to eight attempts for a smoker to be a successful quitter. According to the American Cancer Society, about 44 million Americans have successfully quit smoking. So can you, if you give it a try. Give up smoking for good. Your life and well-being depend on it.

HOW TO STOP SMOKING

There is no one right way to stop smoking, but there are many different methods. I describe a variety of proven techniques that people have used to break this addictive habit as well as anecdotes from real people. If one doesn't work, try another or a combination of them. You should be able to find one or more that work for you.

■ Quit Cold Turkey

As jarring as this may seem, many smokers do quit using the cold turkey method, although it doesn't work for everyone. Those who have been successful offer these suggestions:

- **Set a definite "stop date"** when you are relatively free from stress. Don't select a day when you'll be starting a new job, moving, getting married, or under a great deal of stress. Mark Vaaler, a Florida pulmonologist, stopped smoking using the cold turkey method. "I had smoked all through college and medical school," he said. "When I was about to take my boards for a specialty in pulmonology, I knew it wouldn't be too effective for me to be a smoker while warning my patients to stop. So I gave myself the stop date of 'after my boards.' I took the exams—tough ones, too—smoked one last cigarette, and haven't smoked since."

  Sometimes it takes a scare to quit cold turkey. Bob Orcutt, a security guard, stopped cold turkey after his physician told him he had stage one emphysema. "I woke up the next day—Valentine's Day—and figured it was a good day to stop smoking." It's been over one year and he hasn't had a cigarette.

Often, the stop date is not of your own choosing. My mother, who was a two-pack-a-day smoker (and sometimes had two or more lighted cigarettes going at the same time), continued to smoke even after suffering a heart attack at age sixty-eight. When she had a stroke in her early eighties, she finally stopped smoking and never had another cigarette (although she admitted that she often yearned for one).

- **Share your quit date with friends and family.** By telling others that you have officially set a quit date for smoking, you not only reenforce the date to yourself but you also enlist support from those who care for you. If any of them are smokers, ask that they don't smoke in front of you (better yet, encourage them to quit with you).
- **Become aware of smoking "situations."** Because smoking is a habit, most people have specific times and situations when they automatically reach for a cigarette. Some typical times when the "smoking light is lit," are with morning coffee and the newspaper, when stressed, after lovemaking, after dinner, when you're on the telephone, or when you're feeling lonely or depressed. To help you become more aware of these smoking situations, make a list of those times and situations where and when you are most likely to smoke. You'll become more alert to your triggers and can begin to stave off temptation.
- **Get rid of all cigarettes.** It doesn't do you any good to try to stop smoking if you have cigarettes in your home

"just in case" you need them. You're psychologically giving yourself permission to weaken and have a smoke.
Toss them all out, even those in your secret hiding places
(hat box on the top closet shelf, glove compartment of
the car, the back of the linen closet, etc.). Throw out your
matches, lighters, and ashtrays as well.

- **Keep busy.** When quit day comes, you'll do much better
if you have planned a number of activities to take your
mind off wanting a cigarette. Spend the day at places
where you can't smoke. Go to a movie, the museum, or
the zoo, visit nonsmoking friends, have the grandkids
over, or go out for dinner.

  Keep your hands busy, too. Needlepoint and knitting
are good ways to occupy both hands so you couldn't possibly hold a cigarette. It's not just a woman's hobby,
either. Rosie Greer, the former NFL football player, is
one of the best-known men who needlepoint for relaxation, but there are many others. Get a 500- or 1,000-
piece jigsaw puzzle, do crossword puzzles, read, write letters to friends, go on the Internet, play computer games,
swim or go for a walk, or stroke a small, smooth "worry"
stone, anything to distract yourself from the need for a
cigarette.

- **Avoid usual smoking environments.** Many people
associate a specific environment with smoking, such as
the breakfast table as they're reading the paper. If this is
one of your former smoking environments, change it.
Read the paper in the living room, on the porch, or even
in the bathtub. If you like to have a beer with friends in
your favorite sports bar (filled with cigarette and cigar

smoke), invite your buddies to the house for a beer and
watch the game on TV with plenty of pretzels, popcorn,
and other nibbles to discourage smoking.

- **Stock the refrigerator and pantry.** As you're used to satisfying an oral craving with a cigarette, have plenty of
substitutes on hand, such as pretzels, fruit, cut-up raw
vegetables, hummus, and cheese. Chew sugarless gum or
candy or munch on unbuttered microwave popcorn.
Drink plenty of water, too.

    Patricia Underwood gave up smoking when she was
diagnosed with COPD two years ago. "I'm glad I was told
'the longer distance between me and my last cigarette
means more and more healing,' " she said. "I quit when I
knew I was really in trouble and couldn't breathe and
smoke too. I chose to live. I also used strawberry Twizzlers
as a hand-to-mouth substitute in the beginning."

- **Use visualization.** Practice visualization to help you focus
on other pleasurable situations. Use all your senses to visualize breathing in fresh sea or mountain air, tasting flavors
you haven't experienced since you started smoking, and
seeing yourself with white teeth and hands unstained from
tobacco. Visualize yourself waking up without coughing.
(The process of visualization is described in more detail in
the relaxation techniques section of Chapter 4.)

- **Take advantage of the power of prayer.** For many, the
use of prayer and the belief in a higher power can be
helpful and supportive, especially during the early days
when you are quitting your smoking habit. Nicotine
Anonymous, a worldwide program adapted from Alco-

holics Anonymous, offers a spiritual approach to giving up smoking and encourages you to give up smoking for "one day at a time." For information, check the white pages of your local telephone book or the Internet at www.nicotine-anonymous.org/.

- **Be forgiving.** You may not be successful the first time you try to quit smoking. Don't become discouraged and feel it can't be done. It can and is being done every day by others who also struggle with this addiction. Forgive yourself. You're only human. Then try again, one day at a time.

▪ Cut Down and Out

For many people, however, quitting cold turkey seems too overwhelming. For them, cutting down and then out may be more successful. Tim, a security guard, said he was beginning to find himself breathless when he made his rounds. "I didn't think I could stop smoking cold turkey," he said, "so I began to cut down. Now I'm down to just five cigarettes a day and soon hope to be able to quit entirely."

The trick with this strategy, of course, is not to fool yourself by hanging on to those last few cigarettes and never totally stopping smoking. It helps to make a chart so you can track the decreasing number of cigarettes and have, as with the cold turkey plan, a definite date by which you will no longer be smoking.

▪ Buddy System

As with exercise and dieting, many people find it easier to stay disciplined with a buddy. If you can find someone who is as determined to quit smoking as you are, pair up and help support each other. If you have a craving and feel you may give in and have just one cigarette, call your buddy first and let him or her talk you out of lighting up.

■ Group Support

Many people find it's easier to quit smoking in a group situation, meeting with others who also are trying to quit. This type of group support has long been successful in dealing with other problems, such as alcohol and drug addiction or weight loss, because all the members are either trying to overcome their problem or have overcome it and need the group's social support to continue their success. The group should be nonjudgmental, meet at a convenient time and place for you (otherwise, it's too easy to say, "Oh, it's too late for me" or "I'd have to change buses if I went, so . . ."), and have some members who have been successful and are willing to share tips on how they overcome temptation.

Many organizations offer group programs for smoking cessation. Check your local phone book for the American Cancer Society (www.cancer.org), the American Lung Association (www.lung usa.org), Nicotine Anonymous (www.nicotine-anonymous.org/), Smokenders, and the American Heart Association (www.ameri canheart.org). You also can find an interactive quit-smoking program on the National Jewish Medical and Research Center's Web site at www.nationaljewish.org. It offers information, support, and fun-to-use interactive features to help you quit. Be sure to ask for their booklet *Giving Up Smoking*.

Many other organizations in your community also may offer classes to help you quit smoking. Check with your church or synagogue, a local hospital or health clinic, local college or university, health clubs, or the Chamber of Commerce. As over 70 percent of smokers have tried or are actively trying to quit smoking, it's likely you'll find at least one group program in your community. If not, start one.

■ Individual Therapy

Some people prefer working one-on-one with a health care professional to help them quit smoking. Your physician, the American Cancer Society, the American Lung Association, or the American Heart Association should be able to give you the name of a psychologist, social worker, or counselor who is trained to work with addictions such as smoking.

Talk Therapy

This is just what it sounds like: talking. You'll tell the counselor why you want to stop smoking and, in return, you'll learn nonsmoking ways to handle stress and frustration, and ways to end your addiction. Together, you'll formulate a specific plan to help you quit and to deal with the temptation to light up.

Hypnosis

Hypnosis, a form of concentrated focus, is sometimes used to help people stop smoking. There's nothing to be afraid of with hypnosis. It's not like a nightclub act where people do silly or embarrassing things. You won't do anything you don't want to do.

The therapist, usually a psychiatrist or a psychologist who is trained in treating patients with hypnosis, will ask you to relax and close your eyes. Often you'll be asked to count backward from ten or to visualize yourself slowly walking down a safe flight of ten steps. At some point, the therapist will give you the suggestion that you no longer will want to smoke. He or she may add that you'll find that cigarettes taste bad, have an aversion to the smell of tobacco, or something else that will make you not want to pick up a cigarette. In the hypnotic state, you are more receptive to these suggestions. You'll then be told to slowly "wake up," although you haven't really been asleep. You'll open your eyes and that's it.

Although most people can be hypnotized if they want to be, hypnosis to stop smoking isn't always effective. You still have to change specific behaviors such as not bumming a cigarette from friends, keeping a pack hidden "just in case," or smoking one after dinner or sex.

Telephone "Quitlines"

Thirty-three states have established stop-smoking counseling (quitlines) and more are preparing to do so. According to a study in *The New England Journal of Medicine,* telephone counseling conducted in a real-world setting has helped smokers quit.

When you call a quitline, it is answered by a specially trained counselor. Cessation materials are sent to you, and then you call back to begin the counseling process. For information on how you can access a quitline, call your Department of Public Health or go to www.askjeeves.com and type in, "Where can I find quitline?"

■ Acupuncture

Acupuncture, along with behavioral modification and/or psychopharmacology is now used as a therapy in over 300 private and government-sponsored smoking cessation programs. After giving your medical history to the acupuncturist and being examined, you'll lie down on a table as the acupuncturist inserts extremely thin, sterile, and single-use needles in specific locations of your body. You'll be left alone in the room for fifteen to twenty minutes to allow the needles to stimulate the acupuncture points. Sometimes, treatment will include the use of electrical stimulation of the needles. Then the acupuncturist will return and remove the needles. You may undergo additional sessions as required.

Although experts don't know exactly why acupuncture works in smoking cessation, some speculate that the therapy signals the brain to release specific chemicals that reduce withdrawal symptoms. Others, however, consider acupuncture to have a placebo effect, meaning that it is effective if you believe it will be, but needs to be used in conjunction with other treatment modalities.

Ask your physician or local hospital for the name of an acupuncturist who is trained in the use of acupuncture for smoking cessation.

■ Nicotine Replacement Products and Medicines

There are a number of medicines and medical products that can help you quit smoking and ease withdrawal symptoms. Ask your physician which one or combinations might work best for you. Be sure your doctor knows all the medicines you're taking—prescription, over-the-counter, herbal remedies, illegal drugs, and even eye drops or skin ointments.

Nicotine Patch

There are a number of different types of nicotine patches available. Some are over-the-counter and others must be prescribed by your doctor. Note: *Never* use a nicotine patch without checking first with your doctor, and never smoke while wearing a patch.

You place the nicotine patch on your arm or back each morning, and it slowly releases nicotine into your bloodstream. Eventually, you cut down on the number of patches until you can discontinue their use entirely.

Nicotine Gum

You can buy nicotine gum, called Nicorette, without a prescription at most pharmacies or grocery stores. It comes in mint, orange, and regular flavors. As you chew a few times, nicotine is released into your mouth and absorbed in the blood vessels. You then put the gum between your cheek and gum. Read the instructions on the box and, as with the other nicotine replacement products, don't smoke while you're using the gum. Be sure to discuss the option of using nicotine gum with your doctor before using it.

Nicotine Nasal Spray

Your doctor can prescribe a nasal spray called Nicotrol NS that contains nicotine. You spray it into your nose and it quickly reduces your desire for a cigarette.

Nicotine Inhaler

Your doctor also can prescribe Nicotrol, a nicotine inhaler, to reduce your desire for a cigarette. You hold the inhaler as you would a cigarette, and as you breathe in, nicotine quickly enters your bloodstream.

Zyban (bupropion)

Zyban is not a nicotine replacement product. It's a pill designed to ease your cravings and help you lose your desire to smoke. Zyban is available only by a doctor's prescription. Because Zyban should not be taken if you're on other specific medicines, it is very important that you tell your doctor everything you are taking, whether it's prescription, over-the-counter, herbal remedies, illegal drugs, eye drops, or even skin ointments.

It takes a few days for Zyban to build up in your bloodstream so you should start taking the pill a week or so before your stop date. Ask your doctor how long you'll be taking this medication; most people continue to take it for approximately six months.

If you think that this medication and the nicotine replacement products seem too expensive for you to consider, add up how much you're now spending on cigarettes along with how much you are and will spend on medical treatments for your COPD.

■ What About Weight Gain when I Give up Smoking?

Although most people do gain some weight when they give up smoking, the average is only five pounds. Women tend to gain more weight than men and, for that reason, often go back to smoking to help "control" their weight. It's a bad trade-off.

Here are some tips to keep you from gaining weight after quitting smoking.

- **Remove temptation.** It's just like a weight-loss diet: If it isn't there, you can't eat it. Don't keep a bag of M&M's in your desk drawer, and don't have your kitchen cabinets filled with high-calorie chips. Have plenty of low-calorie snacks on hand to nibble on: fresh fruit, raw vegetables, unbuttered popcorn, pickles, olives, sugarless candy, or melba toast if you need crunch.

Try to recognize what you really want when you reach for food. Does your mouth miss being busy all the time? Chew sugarless gum or gnaw on a plastic drinking straw. Some people miss inhaling; take deep breaths.

Don't keep snacks right next to you so that you can grab them without thinking (as you used to do with cigarettes). If you have to walk from your desk in the den to the kitchen for a snack, often the craving passes by the time you get to the fridge.

- **Reward yourself, but not with food.** While you should reward yourself for not smoking, don't do it with food. Instead, put money you would have spent on cigarettes in a piggy bank and regularly treat yourself with a new outfit, a class you've always wanted to take, a movie or play, or a special dinner with a special person.

- **Slow down to really enjoy your food**. After you quit smoking, you probably will be able to taste things more fully than you ever could while you were smoking. Simple foods—even bread—can taste better. It's fine to spoil yourself a bit with these "simple pleasures," as long as you go easy on the richer dishes. Eat more slowly and allow yourself to enjoy the textures and taste of food. In addition to savoring the taste, you'll give your food more time to reach your stomach so you'll realize you're feeling "full," and can stop eating. When we gulp our food, we eat far more before we realize we've had enough.

- **Don't use food to relieve your jitters.** Withdrawal jitters should last only a couple of days. Don't give in to high-calorie foods or go back to smoking to calm yourself. Instead, sip water throughout the day. Use a straw if it helps you to satisfy the former feeling of a cigarette in your mouth.

Resources to Help You Stop Smoking

American Cancer Society
800-ACS-2345

American Heart Association
800-242-8721
Ask for their stop smoking packet.

American Lung Association
800-LUNG-USA

Centers for Disease Control
Office on Smoking and Health
800-311-3435
www.cdc.gov/tobacco/index.html

National Jewish Medical and Research Center
1400 Jackson Street
Denver, CO 80206
800-222-LUNG
www.nationaljewish.org

Nicotine Anonymous
Nicotine Anonymous World Services

419 Main Street

PMB #370

Huntington Beach, CA 92648

415-750-0328

www.nicotine-anonymous.org/

Offers special programs for those physically unable to
attend meetings.

No matter how you stop smoking, it's worth making the
effort to try, not only to help slow the progression of your disease but also to keep those you love from breathing in your secondhand smoke and damaging their lungs as well.

MEDICATION

In order to treat your COPD, your doctor may prescribe one or
more medications. Some will be pills you take orally, while others may be powders that you inhale. The purpose of these medications is to help you breathe easier and cough less.

Once you're diagnosed with COPD, you'll enter a baffling
new world of medical jargon and terminology that may be con-
fusing, difficult to remember, and hard to pronounce. When it
comes to medication, it's as though pharmaceutical companies
vie with each other to come up with the longest and most difficult name for their products. Apparently lacking imagination,
many of these preparations also have similar sounding names,
making it difficult for patients (as well as the nursing staff) to
determine which is which. What's more, most medications have
two names—the generic name and the brand name.

The following suggestions may help make your medication program easier and safer.

- Ask your physician to write down both the generic and brand names of all the medications you'll be taking as well as how they are pronounced. It's important for you to become fluent in this medical language so you can mention a particular drug by name, rather than saying, "It's a little orange pill with funny corners."
- Make a chart showing what you take, the particular dose of each medication, what it's for, and when you need to take it. (Some medications must be taken on an empty stomach; others, with a meal.) That will help you or a family member remember so no dosage is overlooked.
- Check out your pharmacy's assortment of pill containers. Some of these pill boxes have dividers for each day while others have sections for morning, afternoon, and evening pills.
- If you forget to take a pill, take it as soon as you remember if it isn't time for the next dose. Do not double up.
- Never keep your pills in the bathroom, as the heat and steam can affect them, causing them to become less effective.
- Store your pills in a safe place if you have small children around.
- Never take anyone else's medications. You may think they are similar to yours, but they may be a different strength or could interact adversely with something else you are taking.

- Don't stop taking any medication or go up or down on the dosage without the doctor's permission. Sudden withdrawal can cause serious medical problems.
- Know your medications' potential side effects. If your face feels numb or you have trouble breathing, it could be serious. Call 911 or head for the emergency room of your nearest hospital.
- Always check with your doctor before taking an over-the-counter medication or herbal remedy. They could react adversely with your prescribed drugs, either greatly decreasing or severely increasing the effectiveness of your medication, triggering unwanted side effects.
- If you see more than one doctor, be sure they all know what medicines you are taking, so no one prescribes something that will interact adversely with your medicines for COPD.

▪ Expectorants

Expectorants, sometimes referred to as *mucolytic agents*, are medications that come in liquid or pill form. They help thin the mucus that is clogging your airways and make it easier for you to cough it up. Some brand names of expectorants are Humibid, Organidin, Robitussin, and Fenesin (generic name, guaifenesin). Expectorants are available without a prescription, but you should always get your physician's approval before making your selection.

Water also can act as an expectorant as it dilutes phlegm, making it easier to cough it up. Try to drink eight, eight-ounce glasses of water each day unless your doctor tells you not to because of other existing health problems, such as congestive heart failure, cirrhosis, or acute renal failure, edema, hyponatremia (low serum sodium) and hypothyroidism if associated with fluid retention.

▓ Bronchodilators

Bronchodilators are prescription medications used to relax the smooth muscles of your constricted airways. This dilates or widens them, making it easier to breathe and to cough up sputum. Usually, you inhale the medications through a device known as an inhaler (or "puffer") that delivers a measured dosage of medication with each puff. Your doctor may refer to this type of medicine as your MDI, which stands for *metered-dose inhaler*.

Albuterol (brand names, Proventil, Ventolin, Volmax, etc.), one of many types of bronchodilators, is also available in a solution that can be used with a nebulizer, or in capsules, tablets, or a syrup, although most people prefer the inhaler for convenience. The puffer is used before exercise (for exercise-induced asthma), or as needed. Other bronchodilators include Alupent, Metaprel, Maxair, Tornalate, Bronkometer, and Brethaire.

Know How to Use Your Bronchodilator

It's very important to use your bronchodilator correctly as it is a rescue medication, that is, it's designed to relieve symptoms of breathlessness quickly.

1. Shake the inhaler immediately before using it.
2. Remove the cap from the mouthpiece.
3. Breathe out comfortably and as completely as you can.
4. Holding the inhaler with the mouthpiece down and the bottom of the canister up, put the mouthpiece in your mouth and close your lips around it.

5. Slowly breathe in deeply through your mouth while, at the same time, pressing firmly on the bottom of the canister.

6. Hold your breath for five to ten seconds, which gives the medication time to get into your lungs and begin working, then remove the mouthpiece from your mouth. You may start coughing. That's okay.

7. Breathe normally.

8. If your doctor has recommended a second dose, wait one to two minutes, then shake the inhaler and repeat steps 3 to 5. This gives the first dose the chance to open your airways so the second dose can be more effective.

9. Replace the mouthpiece cap so dust and other particles can't get into it.

10. Rinse your mouth with water after each use.

11. Never use another person's bronchodilator.

If you're still uncertain how to use your bronchodilator, ask the nurse in your doctor's office to demonstrate it for you. It's very important that you use the correct technique in order to get the medicine into your lungs, not just in your mouth. Don't be afraid of bothering the doctor or his office staff. They know how important it is for you to use the right technique with the bronchodilator in order to get the total medication that's been prescribed for you. Once you get comfortable using the inhaler, you'll use it without having to think about the individual steps.

Bronchodilators are fast acting, and for that reason you should always carry your inhaler with you in your purse or pocket when you go out. Your inhaler can't help you if it's on your night table or in the medicine chest. After using your puffer you usually should feel results in as little as a couple of minutes. Although most bronchodilators can be used every three to four hours, always check with your doctor to see how often you can use it. Be sure to keep track of the number of "puffs" you've used so you'll know when the canister is empty.

Be Aware of Potential Side Effects

There may be side effects with bronchodilators, ranging from the common to the more serious. The more common side effects include nervousness, tremor, headache, dry mouth, unpleasant aftertaste, hoarseness, and heartburn, although none of these may occur. Serious side effects may include confusion, chest pain, rapid and irregular pulse, bluish cast to fingernails and lips, and inability to speak. If these serious side effects occur, call (or have someone call) 911 or your local emergency medical service immediately.

Bronchodilators also interact adversely with a variety of medications. Never combine over-the-counter (OTC) inhalants with a prescribed bronchodilator, as many of the OTC drugs contain ephedrine. Do not combine with the herb ma huang, which is a natural ephedrine that acts like epinephrine. Either could interact with your prescribed drug, increasing or decreasing its effect. Always be sure to tell your doctor if you are taking other medications for high blood pressure, digitalis, tricyclic antidepressants, diuretics, or any other prescription, over-the-counter, or herbal remedies.

If you're over age sixty, you may be more likely to experience adverse side effects from drugs because as we age, our liver and kidney functions slow. These organs are the ones responsible for metabolizing drugs, so it takes longer to process and eliminate the chemicals, and the drugs stay in our bloodstream longer. This, in combination with the fact that most people over sixty have more than one chronic condition that requires medication, makes older people more susceptible to experiencing adverse drug reactions (known in the medical world as ADRs). In addition, as many drugs build up in the bloodstream, they can make you feel dizzy and unsteady on your feet, which can lead to falling and possible broken bones.

Note: As with all drugs, never take other people's medication (prescription, over-the-counter, or herbal remedies) regardless of how much it has helped them. Medications never should become a do-it-yourself project. Always check with your physician.

▪ Corticosteroids

Corticosteroids (such as Flovent, Pulmicort, Azmacort, and Vanceril) are inhaled anti-inflammatory drugs that lessen swelling of the airway walls, which also reduces mucus production. This type of drug is available in pill and liquid form. Corticosteroids are often prescribed if airway obstruction cannot be kept under control with the use of bronchodilators alone. Inhaled steroids ease breathing, reduce COPD symptoms, and can improve the effects of bronchodilators on the lungs. They must be used regularly and are used for maintenance, not for when you need immediate relief. (Use the bronchodilator for immediate symptom relief.)

As with the bronchodilator, be sure you've been shown and understand how to use the inhaler for maximum benefit. Always thoroughly rinse your mouth with water after using a corticosteroid to prevent developing creamy white patchy eruptions on your mouth, tongue, and throat, which is a fungal infection known as thrush.

Do not take cough suppressants or sedatives as they can depress your respiratory system and can cause a buildup of pulmonary secretions.

■ Nebulizer

Most metered-dose medications can also be used in a nebulizer, a small device about the size of a telephone answering machine that delivers your medication through a fine mist that you inhale either through a mouthpiece or mask.

It takes a little longer to mix the medication, inhale it, and then clean the device, but it's worth it if you have difficulty coordinating the hand and breathing movements needed for inhalers. Instructions for use and cleaning of the nebulizer come with the device, which you can buy or rent from a medical supply house. Be sure to follow the cleaning instructions carefully to prevent bacteria from building up in the equipment.

■ Antibiotics

Antibiotics are usually prescribed at the first sign of a respiratory infection—an increase in the amount of sputum or a change in its color combined with a low-grade fever. Don't wait to contact your physician in the hopes that you can cure the infection on your own with orange juice and your grandmother's chicken soup. People with COPD have weakened immune systems and can develop serious complications such as pneumonia or breathing difficulties from an otherwise simple chest cold.

Follow these rules to avoid a respiratory infection:

- Complete the *entire* prescribed course of antibiotic treatment even though you feel better.
- Never take a family member or friend's antibiotic when you feel a respiratory infection coming. That prescription may not help you and might make you immune to that particular drug. Particular antibiotics are used for specific bacterial infections. But when you take one that isn't meant for what you have, your body may build up a resistance to it so that drug won't be effective when you do need it.
- Avoid contact as much as possible with those who have colds or respiratory infections.
- Wash your hands often and well.
- Stay away from crowds as much as possible.
- Eat balanced meals and get plenty of rest.
- Maintain good hydration by drinking eight, eight-ounce glasses of water daily unless otherwise directed by your physician.
- Get an annual flu shot and, every five years, an immunization against pneumococcus, which causes pneumonia.

PULMONARY REHABILITATION

Don't be surprised if your physician prescribes a pulmonary rehabilitation plan for you. It is now recognized as an important part of treatment, the "gold standard," for those with COPD.

Pulmonary rehabilitation is an individualized, multidisciplinary program combining education about your disease (for you and your family), exercise, relaxation and breathing-retraining techniques, physical therapy, nutritional advice, emotional support, and the development of coping and support skills to help with lifestyle changes.

Some people who are diagnosed with COPD become depressed and experience a feeling of loneliness and a lack of self-esteem. While that's natural, your pulmonary rehabilitation team can help you through counseling, teaching relaxation skills, and just letting you talk about your feelings. Don't try to "be brave" or "suck it up." They are there to help you feel better physically and emotionally.

According to DeeDee Brayboy, a pulmonary rehabilitation specialist, "Watching these patients get better right before your eyes is quite remarkable and inspiring." The primary objectives of the pulmonary rehabilitation program are as follows:

- to control and lessen, as much as possible, the symptoms and complications of COPD
- to teach you how to achieve the highest level of independence and physical capabilities
- to increase exercise tolerance and encourage participation in recreational pursuits
- to promote independence and self-reliance to improve your quality of life
- to reduce hospitalizations and thereby reduce health care costs

Pulmonary rehabilitation will help you build up stamina for exercise, which in turn will help you breathe more easily. This improvement in the ability even to walk farther without becoming breathless helps you to enjoy everyday activities and is an especially important consideration for COPD patients considering lung-reduction surgery.

Most pulmonary rehabilitation programs are conducted on an outpatient basis and usually run two to three times a week for six to eight weeks. You'll work with a team of health care professionals who are experienced in treating COPD, including physical, occupational, and respiratory therapists; nutritionists; psychologists; cardiorespiratory technicians; social workers; pharmacists; and nurses.

Among the many techniques you'll learn are:

- how to strengthen your respiration muscles so you don't become overly fatigued when breathing
- pursed-lips breathing (exhaling through pursed lips, which makes it easier to empty the overinflated lungs)
- how to maintain bronchopulmonary hygiene so your airways remain as open as possible
- coughing techniques, so you bring up the most sputum with a minimum of effort and fatigue
- aerobic endurance exercises geared to reducing breathlessness so you can better continue conducting a full range of activities of daily living

Patient and family education is stressed throughout the pulmonary rehabilitation program, as you'll need your family's active assistance in many of the procedures you'll learn.

Most insurance companies reimburse for pulmonary rehabilitation if you fulfill specific requirements. Check with your physician to be sure. For a list of programs in your area, contact the American Association of Cardiovascular and Pulmonary Rehabilitation (608-831-6989) or your local chapter of the American Lung Association.

PURSED-LIPS BREATHING

Pursed-lips breathing is an important technique that helps you breathe more efficiently and with less effort. In her article titled "The Importance of Proper Breathing Techniques," Mary Burns, a registered nurse with the Pulmonary Education and Research Foundation (PERF), describes why it's hard to breathe when you have emphysema or COPD and how pursed-lips breathing can help.

Everybody has some air in the lungs even after breathing out as much as possible. This prevents the alveoli, the little air sacks, from collapsing. But patients with COPD may have a 200 percent or larger increase in air trapping.

That extra air compresses the undamaged alveoli, so that they can't work efficiently, and the larger lungs push out your chest walls. Have you noticed that your chest size is larger, or that your bra size has increased? That is why.

Air trapping also causes the diaphragm to flatten. Originally, your diaphragm did about 80 percent of the work of breathing. Now it can no longer suck air in as it tightens and flattens, because it is already flattened out. You are probably working about seventeen times harder to breathe than a person without lung disease.

Now you have to work to get the air out of your lungs. Slow your breathing and concentrate on breathing out: you need to breathe out two or three times longer than you breathe in. If you panic and breathe too fast, or breathe in and out at the same rate, you will cause more air trapping and get more short of breath.

Pursed-lips breathing can raise the oxygen level of your blood as much as, and faster than, being put on two liters of oxygen a minute. Breathe in deeply and slowly through your nose. Breathe out two or three times longer through slightly pursed lips with just a small opening at the center of your lips—as if you are blowing out a candle.

"Don't blow out too hard. If you use too much force, you can actually lower the oxygen levels of the blood. If you can hear yourself exhale, you are working too hard. If you feel uncomfortable doing pursed-lips breathing, or feel that you are working too hard, you probably are. It should feel comfortable and natural.

Also be sure not to breathe in through your mouth before pursing your lips. Breathe in through your nose.

No matter how good your technique is, it won't work if you are breathing too fast or breathing in and out at the same rate or even doing both. It is essential that you slow down and concentrate on breathing out longer than you breathe in.

How can you tell if you are doing effective pursed-lips breathing? Borrow an oximeter from your pulmonologist, or buy one at a medical supply store. If your oxygen levels are low, say 88 percent, with good pursed-lips breathing you will easily blow the numbers up to 93 percent. Really practiced breathers can get their saturations much higher, but 93 percent is a good number to aim for.

For more information about pursed-lips breathing or the work of the Pulmonary Education and Research Foundation:

PERF
Box 1133
Lomita, CA 90717-5133
www.perf2ndwind.org

BREATHING EXERCISES FOR
SHORTNESS OF BREATH (S.O.B)

The natural inclination when you suffer from shortness of breath is to panic, which just makes it that much harder to breathe. But by learning some simple exercises you can retrain yourself to remain calm as you relax, slow your breathing, and begin to use your diaphragm, that flat muscle just below your rib cage and above your stomach, to help you breathe. This will expand your lungs and help to relieve the air that is trapped in your lungs, leaving more room for you to take in fresh air.

When you recognize that you're having S.O.B., stop what you're doing and sit, if you can. If there's no place to sit, lean against a wall. Relax your head, neck, and shoulders. That's important because when you strain to breathe, you start to use your shoulder and neck muscles (known as the auxiliary breathing muscles), and that makes breathing more difficult and much more fatiguing. You don't want to do this. Instead, you need to begin to use the muscles in your diaphragm. Think of a puppet whose strings are loosened. Become a rag doll.

Breathe in through your mouth and out again, using pursed-lips breathing as though you're blowing your hair out of your eyes, whistling, or puckering up for a kiss. Then slow your breathing. Start to breathe in slowly through your nose. Your abdomen should move, not your chest. Don't raise your shoulders. When you breathe out through your pursed lips, your abdomen should go down. Continue to use diaphragmatic breathing until you feel that your breathing is once against under control. Practice this exercise often so you'll feel comfortable using it anytime you suffer from S.O.B.

OXYGEN THERAPY

Although you may be taken aback and somewhat upset if the doctor prescribes supplemental oxygen for you, most people who use it say that daily living is much more enjoyable now that they don't have to struggle so hard to breathe and can exercise longer.

Your physician usually prescribes supplemental oxygen when tests show that the oxygen levels in your blood are low, a condition known as hypoxia. Your doctor will determine the flow rate, how much oxygen you need per minute (also called liters per minute, LPM, or L/M), and when you need to use oxygen (for example, only when sleeping, during exercise, or 24/7, which means all the time). You'll get the actual equipment from an oxygen supplier who brings it to you and shows you how to use and clean it. Be sure to get and post your supplier's emergency phone number in case you miscalculate and are about to run out of oxygen over the weekend or during holidays.

Supplemental oxygen seems to be the only drug therapy that can slow the natural course of COPD and provide a better quality of life. Supplemental oxygen can greatly improve your physical and mental functioning, help you sleep better, and make breathing easier. The use of supplemental oxygen also prevents heart failure if your lung disease becomes severe enough to cause blood to back up into the right side of the heart, enlarging it and preventing its efficient functioning, a condition known as cor pulmonale.

Patricia Underwood of St. Augustine, Florida, has been on supplemental oxygen for more than a year. Her advice: "Don't sit back and assume you can no longer do anything. The trick is to get up and work hard to maintain and improve your health condition every day. Even walking in place for half an hour every day, or even five days a week is enough to keep your lungs working and help out the cardiac as well. I prefer to dance to music, whether it's country or the old rock and roll. It makes the time go by faster for me. I am able to walk farther and with a lot less stress than a year ago since I started this exercise plan. I also try to nap for an hour every afternoon. I take my vitamins and praise God that I am alive and still kickin'.

"I use liquid oxygen and never have to worry about losing power during storms. I also have a portable unit that allows me my freedom." She adds, "My husband and I can still garden, go sightseeing, play Tommy tourist, go fishing, or do whatever we want to do." Recently, Patricia switched to the HELiOS oxygen system, which includes a lightweight (3.4 pounds; 1.5 kilograms) portable tank that fills right from her home reservoir. "I put it in a net backpack (for venting)," she said, "and went out in the yard today and had a good old time working on my plants with both hands free, breathing my oxygen, and not having to pick up and move a portable tank or try to stretch my acres of hoses that are connected to my big tank that is in the house. Even better, it is filled from my tank in the house and lasts for nine hours plus. My husband and I have started fishing again. The ocean air is so good, I can take my oxygen off for hours and still feel great. We go every week now on one of his days off, and I am not only getting plenty of color, but that great ocean air is doing wonders for me. I am so excited about this that I just had to pass it on. There are too many people limited to what they can do because they are still pushing those little carts with the big oxygen tanks, and those tanks are good for only four hours. We need to make people aware that we can still live like other people."

Although you can receive oxygen through a plastic face mask that fits snugly over your mouth and nose and is held in place with a strap that goes around your head, most people use a lightweight tubing called a nasal cannula that runs from the oxygen tank at one end into a two-pronged device that gently fits into your nostrils at the other end. Be sure the prongs face upward. The tubing rests behind your ears or sometimes can be attached to your eyeglass frame. If the tubing rubs against your cheeks, pad it with a small gauze pad. You may have seen nasal cannulas used on patients in television hospital shows. Although it may feel strange at first, you'll quickly get used to the nasal cannula and can eat, drink, talk, exercise, and even enjoy lovemaking with it on.

There is also a third, less commonly used, method used to deliver oxygen, called a transtracheal catheter. A small, flexible catheter is surgically inserted through your neck and into your trachea (windpipe), and the oxygen flows through that tubing. According to Thomas L. Petty, M.D., about ten thousand people in the United States receive oxygen by the transtracheal route. It has the advantages of conserving about 50 percent of oxygen, helping a little in the work of breathing and so may reduce breathlessness, and relieving sore ears and nasal congestion. It is also less noticeable. A transtracheal catheter, however, does carry a slightly increased risk of infection.

Some people use the supplemental oxygen only while exercising or sleeping, but many use it all the time and find that the portable tanks are reasonably light and easy to use, and that the benefits far outweigh any inconvenience. Most individuals using supplemental oxygen while exercising find that it reduces their breathlessness, which in turn allows them to exercise longer, thereby improving their breathing.

You needn't feel self-conscious about using the supplemental oxygen in public. So many people now use supplemental oxygen for a wide assortment of ailments that you shouldn't receive many stares of curiosity, other than possibly from small children who, having seen *Star Wars,* wonder if you're from outer space and hope that you are.

Patricia Underwood says, "I'll stop in the supermarket and show curious children that all that comes out is air. I explain that I just don't have enough so I have to carry some with me. I let them feel the air coming out so they know I'm not making up a story. It's a lot less scary for them that way."

Supplemental oxygen has no taste or smell, and it is not habit forming. Supplemental oxygen can be delivered in three different ways, each with its advantages and disadvantages.

■ Oxygen Concentrator

An oxygen concentrator is an electrical device about the size of an under-the-counter refrigerator. It converts oxygen from the air into a concentrated form until you need it. This type of oxygen delivery is less costly than liquid oxygen and, with a portable system, allows you to move around quite freely. As this is an electrically powered system, you'll need some type of backup in case the power goes out. Notify your electric company that you are using this type of oxygen system so they can put you on an emergency status.

■ Oxygen-Gas Cylinder

An oxygen-gas cylinder is a tank with a regulator, much like that used by scuba divers. Oxygen is released when you inhale and cuts off when you exhale. As the large tanks are heavy, compressed oxygen is usually used while you are at home, although smaller, more portable tanks are also available. These portable tanks provide about five hours of oxygen, so you have to plan ahead if you'll be out longer than that.

▪ Liquid-Oxygen Cylinder

Supplemental oxygen is also available in a liquid-oxygen system. Although liquid oxygen weighs more than its gas form, it is much more concentrated, so the total container weight is less and functional time is increased. While in the container, called a reservoir, the liquid oxygen is converted into a gas that you can inhale. By using a portable liquid system, you can avoid refilling the tank for anywhere from six to twelve hours, depending on the flow being used, so you can continue doing the activities you enjoy. Liquid oxygen is more expensive than compressed gas oxygen, but the freedom it allows you makes the trade-off worthwhile.

As you can see, each of these methods of delivering supplemental oxygen has positive and negative aspects. Your physician will prescribe the type of oxygen you should use according to your needs and your lifestyle and will give you the name of a supplier of oxygen in your area.

▪ Clean and Maintain Your Supplemental Oxygen System

Your oxygen specialist will instruct you in the use and cleaning of the tubing and other parts of the system. If you use nasal prongs, you can wash them with liquid soap as long as you rinse them thoroughly. If you have a cold, change the prongs when your symptoms have passed, just as you change (or should change) your toothbrush after a cold or respiratory infection to prevent reinfecting yourself. It's very important to follow all cleaning instructions carefully to prevent bacteria from growing anywhere in the system and giving you a respiratory infection.

■ Know How to Use Supplemental Oxygen and Be Aware of its Dangers

It's important that other family members or close friends also understand how your supplemental oxygen works and not be afraid of it. That way, if you're not feeling well, they'll be comfortable helping you put on the nasal cannula or face mask and adjusting the flow.

They also should learn what signs signify a change in your respiratory status, as these can mean you're not getting enough oxygen into your system. These signs include your becoming confused, suffering an increase in fatigue, feeling dizzy, or other changes in your behavior. You may not notice these changes as quickly as a friend or family member would.

■ No Smoking Around Supplemental Oxygen

No one (including yourself) should ever smoke while oxygen is being used. Post No Smoking signs to remind guests in your home. In restaurants, sit in the no smoking section. Avoid lighted candles, cooking over gas stoves, and using aerosol sprays while you're using supplemental oxygen. Although oxygen is not explosive, it aids combustion. Materials exposed to flame and oxygen burn more readily and intensely.

■ Flying with Supplemental Oxygen

Although you're permitted to fly with supplemental oxygen, you need to check with the individual airline to learn its particular requirements. Not all airlines offer in-flight supplemental oxygen. You won't be able to use your own equipment, and the overhead masks that are deployed in case of a loss of cabin pressure are not adequate for people who need supplemental oxygen. Most airlines provide oxygen for a fee ranging from about $50 to $150 for each portion of your trip.

Dr. David Claypool, an emergency medicine specialist and medical director of the medical air transport program at Mayo Clinic, offers these suggestions:

- Discuss your travel plans with your doctor.
- When you call the airline, ask for the medical or special services department.
- Ask if they accept passengers who need supplemental oxygen and, if so, what they charge for supplying oxygen during the flight.
- Do they provide masks or nasal cannulas, or should you bring your own?
- Ask how you can transport your own tanks and oxygen generator. Do you check them as baggage, or are they carry-on luggage?
- Do you need to purchase an extra seat for your equipment?
- What documents should you provide and what procedures do you need to follow at the airport and through security?
- Remember that you'll need to make arrangements for supplemental oxygen during layovers and at your destination.
- Don't let the details prevent you from traveling. Although there are a lot of arrangements and phone calls to make, you'll be glad you made the trip.

■ **Do's and Don'ts**

The American Association for Respiratory Care offers these guidelines for people using supplemental oxygen.

- Don't ever change the flow of oxygen unless directed by your physician.
- Don't drink alcohol or take any other sedating drugs because they slow your breathing rate.
- Make sure you order more oxygen from your dealer before you run out.
- Use water-based lubricants such as K-Y lubricating jelly on your lips and nostrils as the oxygen will dry them, but don't use an oil-based product like petroleum jelly or mineral oil because it will affect the tubing and you can inhale oil droplets. Chapstick is okay even though it contains petroleum as it's put on the lips only.
- To prevent your cheeks or the skin behind your ears from becoming irritated, tuck some gauze under the tubing. If you have persistent redness under your nose, call your physician.

For more information about the use of oxygen, check out the American Association of Respiratory Care Web site at www.aarc. org/patient education.

■ **Insurance**

If you meet specific requirements, Medicare, Medicaid, and many commercial insurance plans will cover all or some of the cost of home oxygen. Check with your physician to determine if you qualify.

VACCINATE AGAINST FLU AND PNEUMONIA

Because you have COPD, you are more susceptible to respiratory infections, and they can cause serious complications. That's why it's so important for you to have an annual flu shot, preferably between September and mid-November, as it takes a week or two after the inoculation for the antibody to develop and give you protection. You also should have a pneumococcal vaccine every five years. Researchers previously thought one vaccination was all you ever needed for adequate protection, but they now recommend that the vaccine be administered every five years.

Write down the date you received your pneumococcal vaccine and tape it to the inside of one of your kitchen cupboards. That way, if you switch doctors or your records are misplaced, you know when you had the vaccine and when it is due again.

WHEN IT MAKES SENSE TO MOVE OR CHANGE YOUR ENVIRONMENT

Although it may seem a little drastic, some people decide to move their home in order to live in an environment that is "lung friendly." If your community is highly polluted because of high traffic, factories bellowing smoke and other chemicals into the air, or frequent dust storms or forest fires, or you live in a high elevation that makes breathing more difficult, consider finding a healthier climate.

- Make a written inventory of potential irritants throughout your home, listing them room by room.

- Enclose your bed pillows and mattress in plastic covers so you don't breathe in dust mite debris.
- Use washable blankets or duvets and wash them frequently.
- Don't use the fireplace as it creates smoke in the room, even with a good chimney draft.
- Don't use scented products in the bathroom or kitchen. No perfume either.
- Always use the kitchen exhaust fan when you cook and wash the filters often (depending on how often you cook).
- Change air conditioning filters on a monthly basis and have the coils cleaned and serviced twice a year.
- Buy or rent a high efficiency particulate air (HEPA) filter that removes almost all airborne particles.
- Avoid indoor plants and flowers as they may attract dust and mold. If you use silk plants, dust them often with a damp cloth and not a feather duster.
- Use damp mops to clean baseboards and uncarpeted floors as vacuuming tends to stir up more dust.
- Keep your windows closed so dust and pollen can't blow into your home.
- Love your pets if you have them, but ask someone else to brush them, as pet dander can stir up respiratory problems. If you don't have pets, don't get them (other than fish, perhaps).
- Be on the lookout for other environmental factors that could affect your breathing. Stay inside when the air pollution warnings tell you it is dangerous to breathe the outside air.

SURGERY

■ Lung Volume Reduction Surgery

Lung reduction surgery is also called LVRS or reduction pneumoplasty. In this procedure, about 20 to 30 percent of each lung, the parts that are most filled with disease and no longer function, are surgically removed and the wound closed by stapling. This allows more space for the functioning sections of the lung to expand and for the diaphragm to go back to its normal position so it can work more efficiently. It also reduces the need for the neck and muscles around the ribs to work so hard in the breathing effort.

Who Is Eligible for LVRS

Lung volume reduction surgery was first performed in the late 1950s, but results were poor and the operation was soon abandoned. By the mid-1990s, however, medical technology and anesthetics had improved to the point that surgeon Joel Cooper in St. Louis attempted LVRS again, and this time the results were successful.

Most programs do not accept individuals over seventy years of age, with significant coronary artery disease, who are obese, or who continue to smoke. There may be other restrictions as well, as surgeons are learning that certain patients are better risks than others. Physicians performing LVRS usually require patients to become active in a pulmonary rehabilitation program both before and after the surgery.

Where Lung Volume Reduction Surgery Is Being Done

In 1996, The National Heart, Lung and Blood Institute and the Health Care Financing Administration designated eighteen centers in the United States as sites for National Emphysema Treatment Trials (NETT) in order to determine which is the better treatment for people with severe emphysema: medical management alone (which incorporates medication, rehabilitation, and exercise therapy) or medical management in addition to lung volume reduction surgery.

The United States sites are:

Cleveland Clinic Foundation, Cleveland, Ohio
University of California, San Diego Medical Center
University of Michigan, Ann Arbor
Temple University, Philadelphia
Cedars-Sinai Medical Center, Los Angeles
Ohio State University, Columbus
University of Pittsburgh
Columbia University, New York City
National Jewish Center for Immunology and Respiratory
 Medicine, Denver
Washington University, St. Louis
Brigham & Women's Hospital, Boston
Baylor College of Medicine, Houston
Duke University Medical Center, Durham, North Carolina
Mayo Clinic, Rochester, Minnesota
University of Maryland at Baltimore
University of Pennsylvania Medical Center, Philadelphia
University of Washington, Seattle
St. Louis University, St. Louis, Missouri

In addition, there are twelve major university centers throughout Canada conducting randomized, controlled trials through the Canadian LVR Surgery Project.

University of Alberta, Edmonton
University of British Columbia, Vancouver
University of Calgary, Calgary, Alberta
Dalhousie University, Halifax, Nova Scotia
University of Laval, Quebec
University of Manitoba, Winnipeg
McMaster University, Hamilton, Ontario
University of Montreal
University of Ottawa
Queen's University, Kingston, Ontario
University of Toronto
University of Western Ontario, London

Lung volume reduction surgery continues to be performed at these and additional centers for patients other than those in the study. Speak with your physician if you'd like more information and might want to be considered for surgery.

Complications of LVRS

There are dangers and potential complications with all surgery, and LVRS is no exception. The most common postoperative complication is air from the stapled edge of the lung where tissue was removed leaking into the chest cavity. Normally, a vacuum exists between the ribs and the lungs, enabling the lungs to expand and fill with air. If a leak permits air to enter this space, the vacuum is lost, causing the lungs to collapse, making it difficult for them to expand. There also is a danger of pneumonia or infection, gastrointestinal upsets, stroke, bleeding, heart attack, and even death. At this writing, the mortality range from the lung volume reduction surgery is from 0 to 18 percent. This compares to a 1 to 5 percent mortality for coronary bypass and 1 to 10 percent from lung cancer surgery.

Benefits of LVRS

For many who qualify for this surgery, the potential benefit of LVRS outweighs the risk. Those who have successfully undergone lung volume reduction surgery find that they have less shortness of breath and more endurance, and they are less dependent on supplemental oxygen. The extent of their success, however, greatly depends on their active participation in postoperative rehabilitation that begins the first day after surgery, and, of course, no longer smoking.

Some private insurance companies cover LVRS, subject to specific criteria. At this writing, Medicare does not reimburse for lung reduction surgery other than for those participating in the NETT program.

▪ Lung Transplantation

Lung transplants have gone beyond the experimental stage and are commonly being performed on patients (usually those under age sixty) with severe end stage COPD. The surgery involves taking a lung from a person who has just been declared brain-dead but is still on life support in order to keep the lungs, heart, and other organs healthy. The lung is then transferred to someone who is a "match," that is, of compatible chest size, weight, and blood type to minimize the possibility of rejection. Severity of illness is also a factor. As you can expect, there sometimes is a long wait—the average is eighteen months—for a suitable donor to become available.

As donor lungs are scarce and the procedure is expensive, you have to fulfill specific requirements in order to be considered. Individuals with a history of numerous respiratory infections, recent diagnosis of cancer, or other chronic diseases, such as significant coronary artery disease, may not qualify, nor will those who still smoke.

Before the Surgery

When you are accepted as a potential lung transplant recipient, you'll undergo a number of medical tests including, but not limited to, pulmonary function tests, an exercise stress test, chest CT scan to determine the extent of your lung disease, various cardiac studies, blood work, and even a psychological evaluation. This latter interview is to determine your ability to follow strict regimens of exercise, make all follow-up appointments, remain conscientious about taking numerous pills daily for the rest of your life, and be prompt about reporting any symptoms of infection or rejection. It goes without saying that you agree to never smoke again.

You also need to eat properly and continue prescribed exercise so you are in the best condition possible before your surgery. This prevents your losing muscle tone and aids in your recovery from surgery.

What the Surgery Entails

You'll be put under general anesthesia for this surgery. Be sure to tell the anesthesiologist if you are allergic to any medications, or if you or any blood relatives have had any bad reactions under anesthesia. Some people have a genetic deficiency of certain enzymes that causes prolonged reactions to specific drugs. These people may be difficult to wake up after a general anesthetic.

After the anesthesiologist determines that you are safely asleep, the surgeon makes an incision about six inches under your armpit and removes a small section of your rib in order to gain access to your diseased lung. During this time your blood is rerouted through a heart-lung bypass machine where the blood is oxygenated, just as though it were circulating through your lungs. The anesthesiologist monitors your blood pressure, breathing, and other vital signs throughout the surgery. After your diseased lung is removed, the surgeon replaces it with the donor's lung, sews it into place, and then connects your blood vessels and bronchial tubes. You're then removed from the heart-lung bypass machine and begin to breathe on your own.

After the Surgery

After you've had a lung transplant, you need to take numerous specific medications called immunosuppressants for the rest of your life to prevent your body from rejecting the new lung. The goal is to find the lowest dose of immunosuppressants to prevent rejection of your new lung while at the same time preventing the risk of infection and side effects from the drugs. Remember that there always is a danger of interaction between drugs, even non-prescription, over-the-counter, and herbal remedies. Be sure to check with your physician before taking any medications, even those you formerly considered "harmless."

Antirejection drugs cause you to be more susceptible to the dangers of infections, so you should stay away from large crowds or people who are coughing or sneezing. As bacterial, viral, and fungal infections commonly occur in lung transplant recipients, you also need to report any signs of infection or rejection promptly so they can be treated immediately.

Your physician will give you a timetable for when you need to return for regular checkups and breathing tests. You need to follow this schedule faithfully and continue to exercise as prescribed.

As of July 2002, the one-year survival rate after single lung transplantation was 74 percent, although the three-year survival rate was not as encouraging (60 percent) because of infections (especially fungal) and rejection of the donor's lung. Before a patient is considered a candidate for lung transplantation, death is expected within months, certainly within one year. Most candidates for lung transplant die waiting for a compatible organ. Nevertheless, many people with COPD who have had a lung transplant are enjoying life today, free of supplemental oxygen and able to work and play ten years or more after their surgery. For best results, have your surgery performed at a facility where a large number of lung transplants are done annually.

For additional information about lung transplants, contact:

The Second Wind Lung Transplant Association
300 South Duncan Avenue, Suite 227
Clearwater, FL 33755-6457
888-855-9463 or 727-442-0892
www.2ndwind.org
heering@2ndwind.org

Offers support to patients (and friends and family) considering a lung transplant as well as those recovering from one.

The American Transplant Association
980 North Michigan Avenue, Suite 1400
Chicago, IL 60611
1-800-494-4527
ata@americantransplant.org

Focuses in bringing a patient's perspective to the education, services, and support that transplant patients and their families need.

An excellent book that tells you everything you need to know about lung transplantation is *The Lung Transplantation Handbook*, by bilateral-lung transplant survivor Karen A. Couture. It's published by Trafford and sells for $29.98 ($44.98 in Canadian), plus shipping and handling. You can contact the publisher toll-free at 1-888-232-4444 or on-line at www.trafford.com.

4

What Caregivers Need to Know

You are one of seven million Americans who spend all or part of their day assisting family members or friends who need help to remain at home. Although someone you care for has been diagnosed with COPD, the disease quickly becomes a family matter, not just for a spouse or significant other, but for the extended family as well. And just as the individual with the disease probably has no prior experience in dealing with a prolonged and incurable disease, you, as caregiver, also are likely to feel at a loss for how to cope with the situation. What are the rules? Who picked you to be the captain of this team? How can you go back to the way things used to be, when you had never heard of a disease known as COPD?

Obviously, there are no rules. Each family is unique and handles adversity in its own way. Nevertheless, people who have "been there" as well as health care professionals can ease the way by clearing the path, making you aware of potential pitfalls, and showing you what has worked for others.

A CHRONIC CONDITION CHANGES
FAMILY DYNAMICS

A chronic disease is bound to alter family dynamics in many ways, some major and some barely perceptible, except to one or more of the family members. Quickly, previously normal routines become disrupted. Now you must set aside time for doctor's appointments, pulmonary rehabilitation sessions, and prescribed exercise routines.

If the breadwinner is the one with COPD, he or she may have to slow down or actually retire as the disease progresses. If the partner of the breadwinner has the disease, he or she may have to cut back on hours, use flextime, or rearrange work schedules in order to spend more time with the person who is ill. Finances may become strained; resentments and guilt may grow.

As the disease progresses, the balance of decision making may shift to another family member, causing the patient to feel less needed and the caregiver to feel overwhelmed. You, as caregiver, may find yourself walking a thin line between cheerleader and drill sergeant, as you urge your loved one to eat nourishing food, do the exercises so important in facilitating breathing, and continue socializing with friends and family.

On bad days, when the patient is having more fatigue or difficulty breathing, he or she may become bossy, complaining, and just downright unpleasant, often saying hurtful things and just as quickly regretting them. You must learn to accept that it's the effects of the COPD talking, not your loved one. It takes a great deal of understanding and forgiving. The emotional ups and downs, both yours as well as the patient's, along with additional stress in general, can quickly wear down any caregiver. Part Two details important stress-reduction techniques for both patients and caregivers. Be sure to experiment and find out which ones work best for you.

If the individual with COPD can talk about his or her feelings, family members often find it easier to cope because there is open and honest dialogue. For some families, the diagnosis and the continuing support and education on how to treat the various issues arising from COPD actually draw the participants closer together, making them more accepting of each other and more appreciative of each day they have together. Even if talking about physical problems isn't something you've been comfortable with in the past, give it a try. Your loved one may need to discuss his or her feelings and concerns, and it helps if you open the door.

REBOUNDING FROM THE DIAGNOSIS

It takes a while to recover from the diagnosis of COPD. You and your loved one may have realized that something was wrong for some time, but until the actual diagnosis was made, it was easy to be in denial. "It's only a cigarette cough," or "I'm just out of shape."

But once you receive the diagnosis of a chronic and progressive disease, you're flooded with overpowering emotions as the impact of it all begins to sink in. It's normal to be frightened, overwhelmed, confused, and sad over the thought of the potential loss of your loved one. Your mind grows fuzzy as you try to think of the logistics of finances, your new role as caregiver, and even anger, especially if the patient was a smoker and you had tried unsuccessfully to get him or her to quit. The patient, in addition to the stress of receiving a diagnosis of a chronic illness, may also suffer from feelings of guilt about smoking. You both may feel the loss of control as COPD progresses and begins to take over your lives.

As you and your loved one assume your roles—you as caregiver and your loved one as patient—you may begin to feel alone, as though others in the family have dumped the caregiving role on you. You're weighed down with the extra responsibilities and with trying to remember all the intricacies of medication regimes and the technicalities of the pulmonary therapy sessions. You may be frustrated as you try to help without taking away the patient's sense of independence or destroying his or her self-esteem. You also may find yourself caught in the middle among elderly parents who need you, teenage children or grandchildren who need you, and the patient, who also needs you. Time for yourself? When and how? Resentment may fester as you wonder why other family members and friends don't help more.

You may find that some of your family members are in denial, refusing to accept that their loved one actually has a chronic and potentially life-threatening disease. So they do a disappearing act, leaving all the responsibility in your hands as sole caregiver. In this case, try to encourage them just to come visit, letting them gradually see that although the person is ill, he or she is the same person they have always loved. As they become more comfortable with the situation, ask them to spell you for a few hours. It will give you some time for yourself and allow them to feel needed, which they are.

As your partner's symptoms increase, your social circle may

begin to shrink as friends stop making plans with you because of your partner's disease and the inconsistencies of the "good days" and "bad days." Friends may feel uncomfortable watching their buddy coughing or wheezing, struggling to breathe, or using supplemental oxygen. You begin to feel isolated as you and your loved one find yourselves alone with each other day after day and evening after evening.

It's also normal to mourn plans you had for your future together, the dreams of "someday we'll . . ." Your relationship with your loved one may begin to suffer as you vacillate between worry and resentment, fear and anger. You struggle to deal with loving someone who grows weaker physically while you can only watch and feel helpless. Your sleep, when you can sleep between your stress and your loved one's coughing and wheezing, may become erratic and you stagger through your daytime responsibilities seriously sleep deprived. There also may be a devastating sense of guilt that you are well when the person you love is struggling with this chronic illness.

All these feelings are normal, experienced by most caregivers at one time or another. But it need not all be negative. There are ways to make each day special, to enjoy the positive aspects of your life together. Focus on these strategies. They won't make the COPD go away, but they will make each day more meaningful.

POSITIVE COPING STRATEGIES

Educate yourself about the nature of COPD, the effects of the various treatments, and the long-term effects of the dis-

ease. You need to know what effect COPD will have on your loved one. Read books by experts (see suggested reading on page 223), and find reliable Web sites (listed at the back of this book). Remember that not everything you see on the Internet is accurate. If you are in doubt about some information, ask your physician. Many doctors and hospitals have a patient advocate or a specific individual on staff whose responsibility it is to answer questions. Don't worry about "bothering" the doctor—that's what you are paying him or her for. Ask your questions. Lack of knowledge and concern over what is happening and what may happen next can trigger additional stress.

Become an active member of the health care team (with your loved one's permission). Think of the health care team as a three-legged stool, with the physician and health care professionals, the patient, and you the caregiver as the legs. The more the three groups can work together for the good of the patient, the better the results. If one leg of the stool is missing or wobbly, the stool may topple. That's why it's so important for both patient and caregiver to learn as much as possible about COPD and to ask the health care professional questions as they come up.

Observe the rehabilitation therapy so you can help your loved one do the necessary exercises correctly. Learn the names of the various medications, what each looks like, and what each one is supposed to do, so you can watch for subtle side effects. You may notice them before the patient does.

Keep accurate medical records. Use a loose-leaf notebook with dividers to record (and date) medical instructions, including names of the medications, dosages, and times they are to be taken; names and phone numbers of physicians, pulmonary rehabilitation personnel, and emergency phone numbers.

Also include any information you have concerning insurance, names and phone numbers of people who can help at social services, and copies of your advanced directives. Advanced directives are documents that tell your doctor what kind of treatment you'd like to have, or prefer not having, if you are not able to speak for yourself.

As laws differ in every state in regard to advance directives, you should speak to a lawyer to be sure yours are legal. It is also a good idea to discuss your preferences with your physician while you are able so that, hopefully, they will honor your document.

There are a variety of advanced directives and they may have different names in your state:

- A living will
    The living will document only comes into effect if you are terminally ill with less than six months to live. In it you detail the kind of treatment you prefer in certain situations, whether or not you want to be on a ventilator, have CPR if you stop breathing, prefer hydration, and so on. It doesn't name anyone to make decisions for you if you are unable to do so. That requires another document.
- A durable power of attorney for health care
    This document, also called a "health-care-proxy," "health-care surrogate," or "attorney-in-fact," authorizes you to name the person you want to make health care decisions for you if you are unable to do so. Be sure this individual will listen to your feelings and remember your

views on quality-of-life issues as he or she will have to make medical choices based on your wishes and values, not his or hers.

This document needs to be signed, dated, and witnessed, often by two adults, one of whom can't be your spouse, blood relative, heir to your estate, or responsible for paying your medical bills. Often a notary is required as well. If you select a good friend to be your health-care power of attorney, rather than a family member, be sure to have this document drawn up and witnessed by an attorney so there is no question of who is legally responsible for making decisions for you if you can't. You cannot select your physician or the physician's employee or relative, an employee of the hospital or his or her relative, or someone who is a guardian of your property, unless that person is also your legal guardian. Be sure to give a copy to your physician, your family, and, if they don't live in the same town as you, a close friend.

Remember that these documents are not written in stone. You can change them anytime you wish, although you must go through the same procedures again of signing them and having them witnessed.

To learn the requirements of your particular state, contact your local bar association or medical association.

Communicate so you don't have to guess what's on each other's mind. We all have differing communication styles, and those variations may cause ripples or downright confrontation. One person may want to know everything about COPD, including its downside, while the other may refuse to discuss the illness because talking about the COPD makes it more of a reality, one that you or your loved one doesn't wish to face.

Effective communication can help to reduce stress caused by changes in the family, uncertainty surrounding the illness, and the sense of helplessness and frustration that frequently pops up. Effective communication makes it easier to deal with problems (including sexual ones), while it strengthens trust and deepens love.

Communication is especially important when your family member wants to talk about end-of-life issues. Our natural instinct is to brush off such discussions because the subject is too painful to think about. But advance directives are important for all of us, whether we have a chronic illness or not, to be sure that if we're unable to express our desires later on, they will still be carried out. It's not difficult to write down your wishes, and it will be a relief once you've done so. (They can always be revised if you change your mind.) Just ask your physician or local hospital for an advance directive form.

Chances are, neither you nor your loved one is gifted at ESP, so learn to speak up and express exactly what you feel and what you need. Be honest. Really listen when the other is talking and don't interrupt.

Support your loved one without nagging or becoming overprotective. If you try to do everything because you love the individual, you will take away his or her sense of confidence and self-worth. What you think of as being helpful, your loved one with COPD may consider unnecessary interference and a detriment to independence. Be there to offer help when needed, but not because you can do it faster and with less exertion. It's a little like watching a toddler trying to get dressed. You know you can do it faster and better, but it's important for his self-esteem to do it himself. It's like that for people with COPD. They need to know that they can still care for themselves, even though it may be painfully slow, requiring extreme effort and frequent rests. It's easy to take the ball and run with it when it's handed to you, but sometimes you need to do a little backtracking for the "good of the team."

Live for each day. Make the most of each day by enjoying each other, exploring the wonders of nature, and taking time to say, "I love you." Fulfill as many of your plans and dreams as possible for as long as your loved one's health permits, from traveling to Europe to just sitting on the porch swing and watching the fireflies dance. Remember that tomorrow's an unknown for all of us while today is a certainty. Live in the present.

Speak up when you need help. Many members of the extended family, friends, and neighbors may want to help but don't know how. When someone says, "If there's anything I can do for you, just ask," speak up quickly. Be specific. Rather than saying, "I could use help with meals," suggest, "Could you organize a Wednesday night dinner club where people take turns fixing a casserole or meal, so I know I don't have to worry about cooking on Wednesdays?"

Ask a friend to grocery shop for you on a particular day, run errands, help on Mondays when you change the sheets, or just sit with your loved one, if that's necessary, so you can get out for a few hours. Chances are, the one with COPD is bored with just your company anyway and would love having someone new to talk to or play gin rummy with, or just enjoy having a new face to look at.

Practice self-care. Self-care is self-preservation. Self-care means taking care of yourself first, which often means asking for help when you need respite. When John Donne, English poet and preacher of the 1600s, wrote, "No man is an island," he could have been referring to the fact that we all need to reach out to others for help, building a bridge so others can come to our aid.

■ **Take a time-out**

You can't be a caregiver to someone else if you are sick or unable to help. That's why the motto of the Well Spouse Foundation, a national, not-for-profit membership organization that gives support to partners of the chronically ill and/or disabled, is, "When one is sick . . . two need help."

Tell others when you need a time-out. It doesn't have to be for an emergency reason, either. Getting your hair done, having a massage, enjoying lunch with a friend, wandering through a museum or going to the bookstore to find a new book, or playing a game of tennis gives you a vital change of pace that will recharge you.

Too often caregivers try to tough it out, doing it all themselves until they finally collapse from exhaustion. If you find yourself feeling tired all the time, moody, angry, isolated, resentful, sad, and crying easily, you may be suffering from burnout or depression. Everyone needs help at some time. There's no shame in it and it doesn't mean you're a failure as a caregiver, just that you're human.

■ **Exercise**

You may be ranking exercise low on your list of priorities with everything else that's on your plate, but it's time to move it up to the top. Scheduling regular exercise for yourself is as important for your well-being as it is for those with COPD. A randomized study funded by the National Institute on Aging (NIA), headed by Abby C. King, Ph.D. at the Stanford University School of Medicine, revealed that older women showed significant improvements in stress-induced blood pressure levels and sleep quality after participating in a moderate exercise program as compared to women who received only nutrition counseling. "This is an important study," said Dr. Sidney M. Stahl, chief of behavioral medicine within the NIA's Behavioral and Social Research Program. "Studies show that family caregiving accompanied by emotional strain is an independent risk factor for mortality among older adults. The study gives us some evidence that a self-directed exercise program can reduce stress reactions and perhaps improve the health of caregivers."

So exercise! It needn't be tremendously strenuous. Walking is easy and requires no equipment other than a pair of sturdy shoes. Walk around your neighborhood or at the shopping mall, use a treadmill, or just walk around the house, anything to get your heart pumping and your stress dissipating.

Exercise offers a release from tension because it triggers the production of certain chemicals called endorphins. These chemicals create a sense of relaxation and well-being and act as a natural and healthy tranquilizer. You'll not only feel less stressed, you'll sleep better as well.

■ Get adequate sleep

If your partner's coughing and wheezing keep you awake at night, use ear plugs or sleep in a different room, if possible, so you can get a full night's sleep. Lack of sleep creates exhaustion, lack of energy, a short fuse, impatience, physical ailments, and an overwhelming sense of hopelessness. It can lower your immune system as well, making you more susceptible to infection, which is dangerous for both you and your loved one. There's a good reason the Bible says, "The sleep of a laboring man is sweet." It's because we mend our tired bodies through sleep. It isn't a matter of being selfish. It's caring for yourself, so you can be a healthier and happier caregiver to someone you love.

Be careful about taking drugs to help you sleep. Many of them can quickly become habit-forming. Instead, have a glass of warm milk before bedtime, read, or take a warm bath. Use visualization to quiet your mind, so you aren't making lists of things to do instead of relaxing.

■ Eat properly

Don't skip meals. As proper nutrition is not only vital for the COPD sufferer, it's also important for you so that you can maintain good health. At times you may feel too tired to eat, but force yourself, just as you encourage your partner to eat.

If you don't have time to cook daily, look in your phone book for Meals on Wheels, a volunteer organization providing food to those who need it. You can pay on a sliding scale according to your finances. The supermarket also has a number of fresh and frozen prepared foods you can buy. Be careful about the sodium content, though, as some of them are extremely high in salt.

Although a glass of wine at meals can stimulate your appetite and relax you, be careful not to drink too much. Don't abuse drugs or alcohol.

Join a support group. The purpose of support groups isn't that misery loves company. In fact, if it's a negative, constantly complaining group, you want to get out of it and start hunting for another. Support groups offer social interaction as well as important input from those who have been in your shoes. Caregivers swap suggestions on what works along with warnings on what doesn't. Support groups help you realize that you aren't alone in this struggle with COPD. Because these people have been through the same struggles, they understand the anger, depression, and frustration you may experience from time to time. They are able to offer you encouragement, listen to your frustrations without being judgmental, and offer advice. Sometimes, suggestions from those who are living as caregivers to a family member with COPD can be more helpful than those from a physician who is one degree of separation away from dealing with those problems directly.

Some support groups are available on the Internet. For a list of them, go to http://copd-support.com/links.html. Be careful about Web sites and chat rooms run by individuals, rather than national nonprofit groups, as the information may not be checked for accuracy. An article on support groups in the April 2002 issue of *The Harvard Health Letter* recommends that you look for "a group run by a health professional. They can keep the discussion on track and insure that the medical information exchanged is accurate."

There are also support groups for those with COPD. Encourage your loved one to attend the meetings for the same reasons that they are important for you.

If you're not comfortable going to a support group, talk to a health care professional, such as a psychologist, psychiatrist, social worker, or nurse, or a member of the clergy. Don't keep these feelings—all of which are perfectly normal—bottled up inside. You're not the only one who feels anger, frustration, fear, and resentment along with love, compassion, caring, and devotion. Express those feelings. Talk to someone.

Encourage family members to get involved. Often a caregiver takes over the care of a loved one so completely that the rest of the family and close friends interpret the unspoken message to mean that they shouldn't intrude or get in the way. They back off, leaving the caregiver feeling besieged. Be sure that you adequately express your need to share the responsibility.

Hold a family meeting and ask the others what they'd like to do to help—prepare meals, provide respite, take the family member to doctor's appointments, or just sit and watch a ball game or play chess with him or her.

Encourage younger members of the family to help. That's what being part of a family is all about. Many times we shut out the young people, wanting to protect them from the realities of life. But by letting them help, they learn compassion and responsibility, and they feel needed, which improves their self-confidence. Also it acts as a good warning for them not to start smoking or, if they already do, to stop.

CAREGIVING AT A DISTANCE

With today's mobile society, family members often live far from their loved one with COPD. It makes caregiving more complicated. Shawn Crew lives in Houston, two hundred miles away from her mother who has COPD. "I'm her only child," Shawn writes, "and I do as much as I can from where I live. I find myself having to go to her house more often and having to not schedule anything on the weekends in case she gets worse and I need to leave.

"With the distance thing, I have all the doctors' numbers and they will talk with me by phone to let me know where we stand. The nurses that came a few times spoke with me and, also, my mother has a lot of friends that look after her. We have exchanged numbers, and when I need something done that I can't get down to do, I call and they will help me out."

If you're a distant caregiver, be sure to give doctors and neighbors your cell phone or beeper number so you can be contacted in an emergency.

Contact the hospitals and social services in your family member's community to learn what services they can provide.

Cooking? Housework? Ask your church or synagogue if they know of someone who can fulfill your needs, or check with senior employment services or a home health care agency. Be explicit about the type of help your loved one needs. It may be as little as reminding him or her when it's time to take medications, or it may be more, such as having someone to stay through the night to monitor his or her sleep.

If you need to hire someone to help with light housekeeping or personal care, discuss it first with your family member so you know what assistance he or she feels is necessary. Is it help with bathing or the desire to just have someone there?

When calling an agency, be sure to ask:

- What type of employee background screening is done?
- Is the employee paid by the agency or the employer?
- What types of general and specialized training have the workers received?
- Whom do you call if the worker doesn't come?
- What are the fees and what do they cover?
- Is there a sliding fee scale?
- What are the minimum and maximum hours of service?
- Are there service limitations in terms of tasks performed or times of the day when services are furnished?

When you interview a prospective home care worker, discuss in full your family member's needs and limitations, as well as the home health care worker's experience in caregiving and expectations. Also ask for the names, addresses, and phone numbers of previous employers and be sure to contact them. Understand, however, that people often hedge when asked, "Would you hire this person again?" and may be reluctant to mention negatives for legal reasons.

Be clear about the worker's salary, when he or she will be paid, and reimbursement for money the worker may spend out of pocket for gas, groceries, etc. If the home care worker has a car, discuss the use of the worker's car on the job, insurance coverage for the car, or other travel arrangements.

Be certain to discuss the subject of vacations, holidays, absences, and lateness. Emphasize the importance of being informed as soon as possible so you can make alternative arrangements if the home health care worker is going to be late or absent. Have a list of relatives or friends you can contact to substitute if necessary.

Include your loved one in the interview so you can observe the interaction and determine if the employee's personality will blend with your family member's. When my mother, a lover of the indoors and an avid reader, was recovering from her stroke, the first health care worker we interviewed bounced into my mother's living room, called her by her first name, and rattled off all the activities she had planned, including picnics, bingo, and visits to the zoo. My mother (who had aphasia and couldn't speak) just rolled her eyes. We both understood immediately that this helper wasn't a good fit for her.

Regardless how honest and great you think the helper is, remove any personal papers and valuables, make arrangements for mail to be sent to you, and check the phone bill for unauthorized calls.

Pop in unexpectedly whenever you can or ask a close friend to do so, just to see how things are going and encourage your loved one to speak frankly to you about how the helper is working out.

WHAT THE PATIENT WANTS FROM
THE CAREGIVER

People who are ill often find it difficult to express exactly what they want from a caregiver. They may not want to hurt feelings of those they love by asking them to back off a little, or they really may not know exactly what they want, as it may vary from day to day. That's where good communication skills come into play. Sometimes you don't even need words. Just holding hands conveys love, caring, and understanding.

You may sometimes have to walk a tightrope, helping when the person needs it, but not rushing to help before you know the help is wanted. How do you know for sure? By developing and maintaining open communication with your loved one. If in doubt, ask.

HOW TO FIND CAREGIVING RESOURCES

Contact your church or synagogue or the nearest medical school's department of aging to see if they have services or volunteer committees that can help you.

To locate local caregiving resources such as meal programs, transportation, caregiver support groups, respite care, and other services, check the city or county government sections of your telephone book under Aging or Social Services for the number of your area's Agency on Aging. The Agency on Aging also supports a nationwide, toll-free information assistance directory called Eldercare Locator. You can call them toll-free at 1-800-677-1116 Monday through Friday between 9 A.M. and 11 P.M. eastern time, or go to their Web site at www. eldercare.gov.

Here are other organizations that can help.

Family Caregiver Alliance
415-434-3388
www.caregiver.org
Their clearinghouse offers material on current medical, social, public policy, and caregiving issues. Offers online support group.

National Alliance for Caregiving
www.caregiving.org
A coalition of national not-for-profit caregiving agencies.

National Association for Home Care
202-547-7424
www.nahc.org
A national organization for home health care agencies
with a great deal of helpful information, especially on
how to select a home care provider.

National Family Caregivers Association
1-800-896-3650
www.nfcacares.org
A grassroots organization created to address the common
needs and concerns of all family caregivers.

The Well Spouse Foundation
1-800-838-0879
www.wellspouse.org
An international organization providing support for the
millions of partners of the chronically ill and/or disabled.

CELEBRATE NATIONAL FAMILY
CAREGIVERS MONTH

When you're feeling tired and somewhat unappreciated, pat
yourself on the back. In 2000, November was designated as
National Family Caregivers Month to further recognize the

efforts of unsung heroes (such as yourself) who dedicate themselves unselfishly, day in and day out, to caregiving. But you don't have to wait until November. Celebrate frequently. Then take yourself and your loved one out for dinner, if possible, or order in something special to celebrate.

PART TWO

Living with COPD

5

The A to Zs of Living with COPD

There are two ways of meeting difficulties. You alter the difficulties or you alter yourself to meet them.

Phyliss Bottome,
British novelist, 1882–1963

Once you're diagnosed with COPD, many things in your life will be affected. There are bound to be changes in your energy level, your ability to juggle all your responsibilities the way you used to, and even some of your plans for the future. You'll have to begin to include a sway factor in your daily life, just as architects allow buildings to sway slightly so they won't develop cracks in their facade. These changes are not failures. They're simply new ways of doing things, of altering familiar patterns in order to help yourself adapt to limitations brought about by COPD.

Unlike the movie *Groundhog Day*, every day will not be the same when you have COPD. Some days you'll have more energy and less breathlessness. Other days you may awaken so fatigued that you won't want to drag yourself out of bed. Always be on the lookout for ways to conserve energy, so you have more when you want or need it.

One man who has COPD says, "I consider my daily routine very carefully and, as I know the area very well where I live, I can plan things out. I know where the steps are and inclined pavements as each can provide serious problems. One also has to take into consideration the weather as when it's hot, it reduces my mobility."

A number of the following nonmedical suggestions have been adapted and enlarged upon from hints originally developed by members of the Respiratory Club, a support group for pulmonary patients and their families, at Gaylord Hospital, Wallingford, Connecticut. They come from *Round the Clock with COPD* and are used by permission of the American Lung Association.

APPLYING MAKEUP

- Women usually find that it's less tiring to put on makeup while sitting. If you don't have an actual dressing table, use a card table and hang a mirror on the wall in front of you.
- Collect all of your makeup on a tray or pretty box in front of the mirror to save unnecessary steps.
- Use products that are free of perfume.
- Avoid elaborate hairstyles that depend on extended use of handheld hair dryers and curling brushes. Holding your arm up in the air is fatiguing.
- Use liquid or nonperfumed hair gel rather than aerosol hairsprays.

BATHING

Bathing can be exhausting and wear you out before the day even begins. If you feel weak or dizzy, don't take a bath or shower when you are alone. Ask a family member or close friend to drop by. He or she can read or watch television in another room while you bathe, but be nearby in case you need help.

- If your shower's in the bathtub, get a nonslip rubber mat. You can buy them in most department stores or bath shops. I found a great one (for my grandchildren) in the One Step Ahead catalog. It's big—16 inches by 40 inches—and has suction cups to keep it in place. Call toll free 1-800-274-8440 or go to www.OneStepAhead.com.
- You don't have to take a bath or shower to feel clean. Instead, you can take what used to be called a sponge bath, which is merely washing yourself with a warm washcloth in the bathroom sink. Sit down as you wash, so you don't get breathless or overtired.
- If you want a tub bath but don't feel up to climbing in and sitting on the bottom of the tub, get a slipproof bath chair, put it in the tub, and sit on that. If your tub has a hand spray attachment, you can even wash your hair with only your feet dangling in the water. Bath chairs can usually be found in pharmacies or hospital equipment and supply stores through your Yellow Pages. They can be purchased or rented.
- If you prefer showering, use the bath chair in the shower so you can sit while you shower.
- Install grab bars on the side of the shower and on the

side of the bathtub. Have the installation done by a professional to be sure the grips are secure and won't pull out of the wall or tub when you put your weight on them.

- Use a long handled back brush to scrub your feet as well as your back.
- Be sure the water is warm, rather than hot, to minimize shortness of breath.
- If excess humidity bothers you, leave the bathroom door ajar and use the bathroom exhaust fan, if you have one.
- Many people with COPD use a large terry cloth robe instead of a bath towel. Leave the robe right by the tub or shower so you can easily slip into it. You only have to blot, thus eliminating the effort of drying yourself. It also feels very luxurious.

BREAKFAST

Be sure to ask your physician if it's safe for you to have a grapefruit or grapefruit juice, as there are many medications that should not be taken with this particular fruit. The juice contains a chemical that inhibits the enzyme system, causing grapefruit juice to interact adversely with a number of medications.

- Eat a nourishing breakfast of cereal, fruit, yogurt, whole wheat toast, or eggs.
- If you need help with meal planning, call your local hospital and ask to speak to the dietitian.
- Vary your breakfast menu so it doesn't get boring.
- Never skip breakfast. It really is the most important meal of the day.

• If you feel too tired to eat a full breakfast, break it up into two servings, one when you get up and the remainder around 10 A.M. That also keeps your stomach from getting too full, which will, in turn, press on your diaphragm, making it more difficult to breathe.

BRUSHING YOUR TEETH

• If standing to brush your teeth causes undue fatigue, sit while you brush.
• An electric toothbrush makes toothbrushing less strenuous. Use a little plastic dish to spit into, then rinse your mouth.
• Floss your teeth as you sit as well. Studies have shown that good dental hygiene is vital to protect you from infections, so don't skip this important daily habit.
• If you do have a cold or an infection, get a new toothbrush after it's cleared up to prevent reinfecting yourself.

CLEANING

• Be willing to become more flexible in your standards on housekeeping. You don't need to eat off the floors. That's why we have dishes.
• If you can hire or barter for someone to help you clean, do so and save your energy for other projects that are more enjoyable. PJ, who takes nebulizer treatments about every four hours when she's having trouble with her COPD, says "I do what I can . . . I can dust if I wear a mask. I cannot vacuum because that wears me out too

much. When my honey comes home, he does the things that I am unable to do (vacuum, mop floor, etc.). I usually do all the cooking. I love to cook. When I am having a bad day, he cooks or we order in."

- If you have to use the vacuum cleaner, coordinate your breathing with the movements of the machine. Inhale as you push the vacuum away and exhale as you pull it toward yourself. If possible, ask someone else to empty the bag. If you have to do it yourself, empty the dust onto a damp newspaper so the particles don't fly up into the air.

- To dust, use a long-handled duster or cleaning attachment on your vacuum. As spray wax may be an irritant, use a dust cloth that picks up dust without waxes or sprays. One is the Miracle Cloth that picks up dust like a magnet and contains no chemicals or waxes. I even keep one in my car. They are available by calling 1-800-342-9988 or at www.SolutionsCatalog.com.

- Eliminate as much clutter as you can, without feeling as though you're living in a model house. Bric-a-brac not only collects dust, it also tends to reproduce at a rapid rate until, before you know it, your home is overflowing with china pigs or hippos, crystal bears or bunnies, or cookie jars.

Unfortunately, most of us become used to the mess around us and don't really see it. The junk piles up bit by bit, like tiny, silent snowflakes, until suddenly we realize we're snowbound. To help you see what's there, take photographs of each room. The camera sees it all and can help you determine what you want to stay and what's a squatter, something that sneaked in and stayed because we never noticed it.

- Vacuum books and remove any you have in your bedroom (except the one you are reading now). They not only collect dust but also create mold and other irritants as the paper decomposes.
- When sweeping or mopping, don't bend at the waist. Use a long-handled dust pan to pick up sweepings.
- If possible, remove carpets and use wood or other floor coverings that collect less dust and require little upkeep.
- Rather than bending over to wipe up spills, drop paper toweling on the floor and use your foot to wipe up the spills.
- Use long tongs for reaching things over your head. They're available at most hardware stores, groceries, and medical supply houses. Better yet, get a stepstool on wheels, such as they use in libraries, and step up to get items so you don't have to reach over your head. Never climb up on a chair.
- Use a rolling laundry cart to collect dirty clothes, rather than carrying them to the washing machine. If your machine is downstairs, toss the dirty clothes down the clothes chute if you have one, or over the banister if you don't, making them land into the rolling laundry cart below if your aim is good.
- Take clothes out of the dryer immediately so you can smooth out the wrinkles rather than having to iron them.
- Sit at a table to fold clothes.
- Keep a chair or stool in your laundry area so you can sit when you're feeling winded.
- Sit whenever you can.

COOKING

Although you often may not feel like eating, proper nutrition is an important part of maintaining good health. Staying well nourished (along with exercise) increases your energy level and helps you maintain muscle and bone strength. The trick is not to wear yourself out cooking elaborate meals that you're then too tired to eat.

These tips may help you to prepare a balanced diet without exhausting yourself.

- If possible, prepare a week's menus at a time. When her children were young, Ethel Kennedy is said to have planned two weeks' worth of menus at a time, put them on index cards, and then just rotated them. Try it. That way you know you have all the ingredients for each meal.
- Preplan your meals when you are neither hungry nor tired.
- Utilize convenience foods when desired, but remember that many packaged foods have a high salt or sugar content, which may be prohibited if you're on a special diet. In addition, a high sodium intake can cause you to retain water, which puts extra stress on your lungs. Read labels before you purchase prepared items.
- If you have a microwave oven, use it to reduce cooking time.
- Use a slow-cooking electric crock pot or pressure cooker to make it easy to put foods in and forget about them until you're ready to eat. By tenderizing meat using these cooking methods, you cut down on the energy needed to eat them.

- Use pots and pans that are lightweight so you don't use excess energy just lifting your cooking utensils.
- Keep the pots, pans, and casseroles you use most often near the stove.
- Get organized by measuring and laying out everything you need before you begin to cook, so you don't have to keep hopping up to get an ingredient you forgot.
- Whenever possible, sit at your breakfast table or bar to peel and slice vegetables or to mix ingredients. Bring everything back to the stove on a tray or wheeled cart so you cut down on trips.
- Consider making a double or triple batch of food. Then freeze the excess in meal-size containers that can go into the oven or microwave on days you don't feel up to cooking.
- Always use your exhaust fan when you cook, or make sure that your kitchen has good ventilation.
- If the heat bothers you when you're cooking, use a portable fan. It can cool you off and help to overcome shortness of breath brought on by exertion or stress. It's also useful for blowing away all sorts of odors.
- Bake in pretty casseroles that can go directly from the oven or microwave to the table.
- When tidying up after a meal, assemble all items that need putting away in the refrigerator on a tray. Then put them away one at a time.
- To avoid having to scrub pots and pans, pour a little dishwasher detergent in and add hot water, then let the pots soak for an hour or so. The stuck-on food will easily wash away.

- After washing dishes, put your most used pots and pans back on the stove and leave them there. Rather than putting away your dishes and silverware, reset the table for your next meal.

- Sort through your kitchen appliances, utensils, and pots and pans. Give away any that you haven't used within the last year. You'll not only be amazed how much more room you have in your cupboards, you also won't have to expend energy lifting up one or more bowls or pans to get to the one you want to use.

- Don't be tempted to buy supplies in the extra-large, economy size. Even though you may save money, the packages are usually extremely heavy to lift and you'll have to strain every time you try. If you feel you must go for quantity, get a good supply of smaller disposable plastic containers and divide the supplies into more manageable sizes, marking each container carefully. The only exception to repackaging is cleaning supplies. They should never be removed from their original containers. Even if carefully marked, these products could be mistaken for something edible or drinkable, if not by you, by a child or other family member.

- Use grocery delivery services if your area has them or hire a responsible high school student to shop and deliver your groceries for you. The extra charge is balanced by the energy you will save for something more fun, and you will have helped to teach a young person a great deal about responsibility and helping others.

- Go through your kitchen junk drawer while you're sitting and talking on the phone. It's a good time to toss ball-point pens that don't work, gadgets you don't use, and rubber bands you've collected from the newspaper. Clutter causes you to waste energy.

DEPRESSION

Depression is an insidious disease. It slowly sneaks up on you like extra pounds. And not only on you. When one family member is depressed, it often spreads throughout the rest of the family like a creeping, but steady, lava flow. That's why depression is often considered to be an "infectious disorder."

"I hadn't realized how depressed my son and I had become living with my husband's depression," a friend said, "until I took my son to the pediatrician for his precollege check up. We sat there, passive and secretly relieved to be out of the house, when a woman walked in with two identical twin boys about nine months old. They were adorable. We couldn't help smiling. Then a couple came in with their fifteen-month-old little girl. She looked at the two little boys, sitting like the proverbial two peas in a pod on the floor in their car seats. The little girl looked at one face, then the other. Then back to the first. The expression on her little face at seeing two babies that she, still a baby herself, recognized as identical, was priceless. We all laughed. It felt so good. My son and I couldn't stop laughing and watching that little girl stare at those two babies and how they stared back. We hated to hear the nurse call my son's name so that we had to leave."

You may not even realize that you are depressed. You just feel tired and sad, have aches and pains and a pervading sense of hopelessness, and seem to have lost your zest for life. You withdraw from social activities because it's just too much effort. "It's because of my COPD," you tell concerned family members and friends. And to a degree, you may be right. Many of the symptoms of depression also may be effects of COPD, such as significant weight loss, sleeping all the time (or insomnia), extreme fatigue or loss of energy, feelings of worthlessness or excessive guilt (because you were a smoker), or an overwhelming sense of sadness. These as well as recurrent thoughts of death or suicide all point to a possible diagnosis of depression.

Of course, you have every reason to feel anxious or depressed at times. Your COPD is a progressive and chronic condition and one that will change your life from now on. What's more, there may be biological reasons for depression, including hormonal changes in your body due to the ineffectiveness of your lungs' functioning and the fact that your brain may not be getting enough oxygen from your blood. But there's a difference between experiencing blue periods and having clinical depression, and to make that distinction you need the services of a mental health specialist—a psychologist, psychiatrist, or clinical social worker.

Psychiatrist Eric Pfeiffer, director of the Suncoast Gerontology Center, University of South Florida in Tampa, admits that detecting depression can often be very difficult. A depressed person's behavior may vary depending on whom he or she is with at a particular time. "Sometimes a depressed person can only carry out one role," Pfeiffer said. "That is, a man might function satisfactorily at work but be nonfunctional at home. At the office, his coworkers think he's fine. Yet his wife complains that he collapses when he gets home, sits in front of the television, never talking, and is negative about everything and everybody. The man's peers at work can't understand what the wife is complaining about."

But don't think you're the only person with depression. Depression is an equal opportunity disease and almost nobody escapes from it at some point in life. They either suffer from it personally or try to cope with a family member who is afflicted. It is the most common biological disorder seen in psychiatry today. Scores of actors, writers, and politicians now openly admit doing battle with it. So there's no reason to feel embarrassed if you suspect that you or someone in your family is suffering from depression.

■ Get Professional Help

You can't fight depression by yourself. It seldom just goes away on its own. Tell your physician if you feel you may be suffering from depression. There are many forms of effective treatment, including antidepressant medication and short-term psychotherapy (or talk therapy). Medications include tricyclics such as Elavil and Tofranil, serotonin inhibitors like Prozac, and monoamine oxidase (MAO) inhibitors such as Nardil and Marplan.

Get professional help. If you entertain thoughts of suicide or that your family would be better off without you, get help immediately. Don't wait, figuring those feelings will magically go away. Ask your doctor for the name of a psychologist, psychiatrist, or clinical social worker, or see a member of the clergy.

■ Never Underestimate the Power of the Mind

Although you can't cure depression on your own, you can talk yourself into a sense of calmness by bolstering your happiness potential. Each day, promise yourself that you'll banish negative thoughts, worries about things not in your control to change, and guilt. Focus on those things that make you smile. The secret is simple. No one can think of two things at once. By focusing your mind on happy thoughts, you can't think about the negative or depressing ones.

More than twenty years ago, I was diagnosed with breast cancer. I wasn't shocked by it; the offending lump had felt different from all the others I had previously experienced. Somehow I sensed that it was malignant this time. I had a biopsy under a local anesthetic. The physician confirmed that, to his surprise, my "cyst" was a malignant tumor. My husband and I went home to weigh my surgical options.

Later, that afternoon, I felt well enough to go to the neighborhood fish market to buy some fish for dinner. I was wrapped up in my thoughts as I paid the owner and took my fish. "Have a wonderful, beautiful day," he said, as he always did.

My first thought was, "A wonderful, beautiful day? I just found out I've got cancer!" Then I thought a minute and a big smile forced its way onto my face. He was right. It was a wonderful, beautiful day. I was still around to enjoy it. I had five great kids, a wonderful, caring husband, and a writing career I loved. How lucky I was to be alive.

I've thought about that day often. The fishmonger's comment crowded out any negative thoughts I had carried around after receiving the diagnosis. I couldn't be depressed because my mind was filled with thoughts of wonderful, beautiful things. That doesn't mean, of course, that I was never depressed. I cried in my husband's arms many times; I cried alone, too. I was afraid and angry. I had written about breast cancer; I wasn't supposed to have it.

But when I felt blue, I did think about the man at the fish

store and what he had said. It made me smile then; it still does. Ten years later—far too long to have waited—I went back and thanked him for cheering me up on that scary day.

■ What You Say to Yourself

I once had a teacher who said, "He who talks to himself is a fool." I think she was talking about those who chatted in class or who mumbled aloud during test-taking time. But other than that, she was mistaken. Positive self-talk is very important and keeps you feeling optimistic and upbeat. Unfortunately, many of us walk around telling ourselves negative things about those around us and even about ourselves.

Contrary to myth, words *can* hurt you, and many of our thoughts are filled with criticism from family members from our youth. These negative thoughts can not only destroy our self-esteem but also stifle any opportunity for overcoming the problems inherent in living with COPD. Unfortunately, most people tend to focus in on negatives and then wonder why they are tired, depressed, and sad.

But when we talk to ourselves in a positive way, what experts call "self-verbalizing," we can raise our self-esteem and remind ourselves that we are likable, resourceful, worthwhile, deserving, caring, and a number of other affirmative attributes even though struggling with a chronic illness. According to Shad Helmstetter, author of *The Self-Talk Solution,* "Self-talk is a means of consciously reprogramming your subconscious mind through the use of specifically worded phrases of *self-direction.*" He describes how self-talk can help us reduce stress, keep exercising, stop smoking, and even lose weight. But first we have to consciously think positively about ourselves.

This exercise may be difficult initially because most of us were raised to be modest about accomplishments and to downplay successes. Thankfully, however, times have changed and we can, too. Begin by making a list of your positive points. Don't just think about them. Actually write them down. Include your special qualities such as liking animals, being artistic, being able to fix anything, or having a good sense of humor. Ask your partner or friends to help you list more positive points (and do the same for them). Paste the list on the mirror in your bathroom or bedroom so you can read each point aloud and not just think it.

What does this self-talk accomplish? It helps you to believe in yourself, boosts imagination and creativity, and gives you a positive pat on the back—and the encouragement to live a full life even with your disease and to help others along the way.

If you're trying to achieve your maximum happiness potential, it might be helpful to consider adopting the following suggestions:

- Believe that you deserve to be happy, even as you struggle with the effects of COPD.
- Surround yourself with happy, positive people; happiness is contagious.
- Write down three things that make you happy. Focus on them when you feel depression creeping up on you.
- Allow your guilt to fly away. You can't change the past. What happened, happened. But you can change the way you perceive today.
- Give yourself the gift of time. Recharge and soothe your spirit through exercise, meditation, listening to music, or

whatever gives you pleasure. If work makes you feel alive, try to continue at your job as long as you can or find part-time work that is fulfilling.

- Practice the relaxation techniques mentioned later in this chapter and make them part of your daily life.

Remember to smile. It not only makes you happier, it also makes people smile back. And as the fishmonger told me, "Have a wonderful, beautiful day."

DRESSING

Many people feel that finishing dressing before breakfast gets the day off to a good start. Others find that dressing first wears them out, so they are too tired to eat breakfast. Try it both ways and see what works better for you.

- Don't wear anything that restricts your chest and abdominal expansion. For this reason, avoid tight bras, belts, and foundation garments (we used to call them girdles). If you must choose between style and comfort, opt for comfort every time. Women who have given up wearing a bra may find camisoles a comfortable and pretty substitute.
- Avoid socks and stockings that have elastic bands that may bind the leg and restrict circulation.
- Shoes that slip on take less bending than those with shoelaces or even those with Velcro.
- Men may find that suspenders are more comfortable than a belt.

- Most women, whether they have COPD or not, acknowledge that slacks and socks are much easier to put on than struggling with panty hose.
- Avoid tight ties or neck scarves. An open neck is much more comfortable.
- Many people with COPD are bothered by extremes of temperature and find that cotton underclothing is more comfortable than synthetic. You can usually find them in department stores, and some nationwide mail order houses carry complete lines of cotton undergarments including "vests" for women.
- As sweaters can be awkward to put on and take off, consider using a large shawl. Today shawls come in a variety of fabrics including wool, cotton, cashmere, and even linen.

DRIVING

- As with other activities, coordinate your breathing with your movements. Inhale and, as you exhale, step into the car.
- Rest before starting the motor.
- If possible, drive a car with automatic gearshift and power steering.
- Try to schedule your driving so it's before or after rush hour. It's less hectic and you'll breathe fewer gas fumes.
- Consider getting a handicap parking sticker or license plate so you don't have to walk as far to stores and back from them with packages in your arms. Your physician needs to prescribe it through the Division of Motor Vehi-

cle Registration. In some states, members of AAA can apply (with the doctor's prescription) through that organization.

EATING

Easy breathers might think it would be great to be told that they had to eat more so they could maintain a weight normal for their height. But it's a serious matter for those with COPD. For some yet unknown reason, 25 percent of those with COPD have difficulty maintaining their normal weight and need to boost their daily caloric intake. Researchers speculate that the weight loss might be because one burns more calories in the struggle to breathe or because the fatigue that overcomes a person with COPD just makes the simple act of chewing too much of an effort.

It also may be that breathlessness and increased sputum production put a damper on one's appetite. It's hard to catch your breath and eat, too. It seems easier not to bother.

■ Why Eating's Important

Eating is far more than just ingesting food. You need to maintain a proper balance of nutrients—proteins, carbohydrates, and fat—if you're going to improve your endurance and boost your immune system so you aren't so susceptible to infection. When you're underweight, you may chill easily and tire quickly. If you're losing weight, you're also losing muscle tone, and that's a problem because your breathing muscles need to be strong. You use ten times more energy to breathe than does someone without COPD. Proper nutrition and exercise can help to strengthen those muscles.

■ **What to Eat**

To increase your weight in a healthy way and to maintain it, you used to be advised to follow the food pyramid guidelines developed in 1992 by the U.S. Department of Agriculture (USDA) and the U.S. Department of Health and Human Services. But recently, experts are turning that pyramid on its head. Dr. Walter Willett and his colleagues at the Harvard School of Public Health now recommend limiting carbohydrates to whole grains and eating no more than two to three servings a day, and replacing red meat with beans, nuts, and fish (i.e., the "good" proteins).

Willett emphasizes whole foods rather than processed foods; cautions limited use of white bread, white rice, pasta, and sweets; and agrees with your mother that you should eat your vegetables—lots of them. His definition of "good fats" is plant oils such as those found in nuts and vegetables. At the base of Willett's Healthy Eating Pyramid is "daily exercise and weight control."

Keep these points in mind as you plan your menus.

- If there's a choice between a low-calorie food and a high-calorie food, select the one with more calories, such as avocados, sweet potatoes, whole wheat bread, and peanut butter.
- Ask your doctor or the hospital's registered dietitian to advise you on the use of nutritional supplement options such as canned drinks that are especially formatted to provide a nutritional balance. Unfortunately, according to the American Institute for Cancer Research, only one in four American medical schools offers any form of

nutritional training to their medical students. For that reason, you may be better served by checking with a registered dietitian or nutritionist at your local hospital.

- Eat vegetables, either raw or cooked. Recent studies show that antioxidant-rich vegetables contain vitamins and compounds called phytochemicals that help to reduce airway stress and slow tissue damage.

- Drink eight, eight-ounce glasses of water each day, unless your doctor tells you not to. This fluid will keep you hydrated, will moisten your mucous membranes, and can thin the mucus secretions and make them easier to cough up. This is especially important if you use supplemental oxygen, which tends to dry up the mucous membranes of your airways. Do check with your doctor, however, as some coexisting conditions may require limiting your liquid intake.

- Ask your physician if you can have either a small glass of wine, one mixed drink, or a glass of beer before dinner, if it doesn't interact with your medicines. Alcohol not only adds calories, it also can stimulate appetite. Don't drink more, however, as these calories are empty calories without nutritional benefit.

- When adding fats to your diet, select vegetable oils (especially olive oil) rather than animal fats found in meat and dairy products. Olive oil contains mostly monounsaturated fat that may help to calm airways. Omit coconut and palm oils usually found in commercial baked goods such as cookies and cakes.

- Eat foods high in protein to help you build and repair your muscle and bone strength. These foods include (but are not limited to) chicken, beef, pork, fish and shellfish, nuts, eggs, dairy products, and beans.

- If you take steroid pills regularly to decrease swollen airways, be aware that the medication could interfere with the way the body uses certain nutrients. For that reason, you should eat foods high in calcium, such as dairy products, to prevent osteoporosis.

- Don't write off beef or lamb as being too hard to chew. By using a slow cooker or pressure cooker, you can stew the meat with little effort. Add frozen veggies and you've got a meal or two without working too hard in the kitchen.

- According to research done in the Netherlands, vitamin C and citrus fruits rich in vitamin C improve lung function.

- To add extra calories to your meals:
  - mix sour cream into your mashed sweet potatoes and melt over vegetables
  - dot your fish, chicken, or meat with a teaspoon of butter just before eating
  - spread peanut butter or cream cheese on your whole wheat toast or bagel, then add jam
  - spread mayonnaise on sandwiches and in egg salad and tuna salad. (My daughter dips her french fries in mayonnaise instead of catsup.)
  - add cheese to cooked vegetables, sandwiches, and salads, and eat as a snack

- Make your bedtime snack custard, cheese, nuts, or a sandwich, but eat the treat at least two hours before retiring so you don't have acid reflux, a condition also known as GERD, in which stomach acid backs up into the esophagus causing what is commonly known as heartburn, as well as potentially more serious conditions.

- If you have medical conditions in addition to COPD, you may have specific dietary restrictions. Ask your doctor or a registered dietitian to help you plan meals around those limitations.
- In addition to eating a well-balanced diet, you may need a multivitamin, although vitamin pills don't take the place of the nutrients you need from food you eat. Ask your doctor to recommend a good multivitamin.
- Be sure to include fiber in your diet to prevent constipation. Fiber comes from vegetables, bran, dried and fresh fruit, beans, sweet potatoes, whole wheat bread, and whole wheat or bran cereal. Increase your fiber level gradually so you don't feel gassy, which makes breathing more difficult. If you feel you're eating enough fiber and drinking water frequently, but still have problems with constipation, ask your doctor for the names of suitable over-the-counter medications.

What Not to Eat

- Avoid empty-calorie foods such as coffee, tea, and candy that only fill you up without offering any real food value. Caffeine also acts as a diuretic and may interact with some medications you're taking.
- Avoid salty foods, which contain too much sodium that can cause you to retain fluids. That makes breathing more difficult. Salty and spicy foods also can make you cough more. In experimental studies, a high sodium

intake was shown to increase bronchial hyperresponsive-
ness. Check labels on canned soups, frozen dinners, and
salad dressings and select those that are low in sodium.

- Don't put the salt shaker on the table. It's too tempting
  to use it even before tasting what you're about to eat.

- When you are having extra trouble breathing, avoid
  dairy products such as milk, cheese, and butter, as they
  tend to produce more phlegm.

- Although a glass of wine or beer can stimulate your
  appetite, too much alcohol is a depressant and can fill you
  up with empty calories, keeping you from eating the
  proper balance of food your body needs.

- Avoid foods that make you gassy or make you feel bloated.
  This can trigger acid reflux or cause your stomach to press
  against your diaphragm, which makes breathing harder.
  Those foods vary from person to person, and what makes
  one person very gassy may not bother another. You'll have
  to experiment, keeping a food diary to determine which
  foods bother you. Generally, however, the common offending foods include cabbage, brussels sprouts, melons,
  cucumbers, raw onions, beans (especially baked beans),
  spicy foods, and peppers.

- Avoid carbonated drinks because they also can cause gas.
  In addition, they fill you up and offer no redeeming food
  value.

- Don't drink a lot of water before or as you're eating
  because it will fill you up.

- Don't drink grapefruit juice or eat grapefruit without
  checking with your doctor, as grapefruit interacts with
  various medications.

■ **How Much to Eat**

It's hard to eat too much when you have COPD because you may not have much of an appetite and you may be too fatigued to feel like eating. You also may be suffering from depression that can decrease your interest in food. Here are some tips that may help you get enough calories in so you can keep your weight up to its proper amount.

- Graze throughout the day. That is, eat five to six mini-meals throughout the day—a banana and dish of custard midmorning, peanut butter sandwich midafternoon, and so on. That way you won't get too full.
- If eating fatigues you or if it's difficult to eat because your dentures don't fit properly, choose foods that are easier to chew such as stewed meats and chicken, fish, and cooked vegetables. And see your dentist.
- Make mealtime pleasant. Much of our appetite begins with the senses, especially the eyes. Set a pretty table and use colorful place mats or dishes, even if you're alone. Play soothing background music during mealtime rather than listening to the news with all the stress it conjures up. It takes a lot of effort for someone with COPD to eat, and eating under stress adds extra difficulty.
- Use dinner-size plates but with smaller helpings. Too much food can be overwhelming when you don't have much of an appetite to begin with.
- Use sturdy paper plates if washing dishes tires you. The nutrition from what you eat is important, not what you serve the food on.

- Vary the color of foods you serve, such as sweet potatoes, green beans, and broiled chicken breasts. A multicolored menu is much more appetizing than a monochromatic one of mashed white potatoes, white beans, and white fish.
- Try not to eat alone. Pleasant company helps stimulate your appetite even if you can't make the extra effort for conversation. If you must dine solo, read a book or watch a favorite TV show. Again, try to avoid watching the news while you eat, as it is usually unpleasant.
- Many restaurants now prepare foods to go. You simply call ahead, order, then go pick it up. If you don't have transportation, ask what they charge to deliver.
- If family members or friends ask what they can do to help, whip out your grocery list. Food shopping is tiring even when you're 100 percent healthy, so welcome the opportunity to let others do it for you. Let them know your food preferences and describe what you want in as much detail as possible.

When to Eat

- Follow the above suggestion about grazing throughout the day.
- Eat your biggest meal at noon.
- Perform your breathing exercises an hour before mealtime so mucus is less likely to interfere with your eating.
- Take a short nap before mealtime.
- If you're the cook, buy prepared meals (watch the sodium content) or make a double batch so you can use it for more than one day. Then nap before it's time to eat.

- Wait at least two hours after eating before lying down. Lying down right after eating increases your risk of heartburn and acid reflux.
- Eat after exercising because you're less likely then to have reflux and have less difficulty with your breathing. If, however, you feel you need to eat something to "keep your strength up," have a small snack before exercising or doing anything that requires additional energy.

Although there is no specific diet recommended for those with COPD, a balanced diet is vital. You must take seriously the need to keep your weight up because when you lose weight, you also lose muscle strength.

And remember, if you're used to having a cigarette after eating, don't do it. Smoking will only make you sicker. See Chapter 3 for tips on how to stop smoking.

■ How to Lose Weight

Some people, especially those with chronic bronchitis, struggle with being overweight, if not obese. Extra weight not only increases the effort your heart and lungs must expend trying to supply oxygen to all areas of the body but also makes it difficult for your lungs to expand fully because the excess fat in the abdominal area pushes against the diaphragm. Being too heavy puts an added burden on already weakened lungs struggling to take in additional oxygen needed for the heavier weight and expelling the excess carbon dioxide. The extra weight makes it more difficult to breathe.

That's what happened to seventy-five-year old COPD patient Francis W. Birch. He's a retired lawn maintenance man, although he still regularly mows his own lawn, now with a self-propelled mower. "It's the last thing I'll give up," he said in a telephone interview, adding that "there are right and wrong ways to mow a lawn. You don't want to mow it the same way each time. It isn't good for the grass." Then he admitted that he reluctantly needed to pay someone to clean out behind the bushes. "I've gained weight recently," he said. "My stomach's gotten big. When I try to bend down to clean out the leaves, I get too winded."

It's the same principle pregnant women experience. When the abdomen gets too big, it's difficult for the diaphragm to expand adequately to bring in air. That's why expectant mothers often find themselves feeling breathless. When you have COPD, however, there's no delivery date that's going to make that tummy go away. You need to lose weight to help reduce the burden on your pulmonary system.

Lose Weight Safely

- Check with your doctor before signing up for any weight-loss plan.
- Don't grasp at the quick weight-loss schemes. If they promise that you'll lose more than two pounds of weight a week, they aren't safe.
- Continue to eat a balanced diet.
- Don't take *any* diet reduction medications, pills, liquids, etc., without checking with your doctor first.
- Include some exercise in your weight-loss plan.
- Be patient. One and a half or two pounds a week is a safe loss.

- Go for five. Rather than looking at having to lose thirty pounds overall, visualize it as one five-pound victory six times. It's easy to think of what five pounds is—visualize five pounds of sugar or flour, five pounds of dog meal or cat litter, etc. It isn't as overwhelming as facing thirty or more pounds.
- Read food labels to determine calories and fat grams.
- Think of yourself as a person who eats in moderation, not as someone who is dieting.
- Watch portion size. A two to three-ounce serving of meat, turkey, or fish is the size of the palm of your hand. Most obesity is caused by supersize food and drink servings. Think small.
- Reward yourself for small successes, but not with food.
- Stop feeling that you must clean your plate: It doesn't help starving children anywhere regardless what your mother told you.
- Drink eight, eight-ounce glasses of water a day, one of them ten minutes before you sit down to eat (unless told otherwise by your physician).
- Do not skip breakfast.

Just as you need to eat more calories in order to gain weight, the reverse is true in order to lose weight. But before you can eat less, you need to know what you are eating now.

Keep a food diary. Once you start keeping a food diary, you'll be surprised at how much you eat without thinking about it—a handful of nuts, a soft drink, a candy bar, etc. They all add up. Commercial weight-loss organizations like Weight Watchers that teach people how to lose weight while eating regular food always suggest keeping a food diary and recording every bite that you eat.

A food diary doesn't have to be fancy. You can record it in a small notebook or on your computer, or make a graph, such as illustrated below:

FOOD DIARY

(Record everything you eat as well as the portion size)

	Sunday	Monday	Tuesday	Wednesday	Thursday	Friday	Saturday
Breakfast							
Snack							
Lunch							
Snack							
Dinner							
Snack							
Water*							

* put a check mark for each glass of water you drink

Keeping a food diary keeps you focused and helps you make smart choices. It puts you in charge and in control of your eating. When you immediately write down what you've eaten, you have an accurate record. Memory is selective and uncertain. Your subconscious may help you to forget the second brownie or the plate of french fries. A Chinese proverb says it best: "The palest ink is better than the best memory."

Be honest in your food diary. If you cheat, you're only hurting yourself and your weight-loss plan. It might help if you jot down triggers that led to overeating. Were you bored? Angry? Frustrated? Stressed? Did you eat as a substitute for smoking? If the answer to this is yes, please don't consider going back to your smoking habit. Smoking is far worse for your COPD than your extra weight.

Set a start date. Just as smokers need to set a definite date when they'll stop smoking, those who are overweight need to set a specific time when they'll get serious about weight loss. Don't pick a date that is stressful for you or where you are doomed to failure, like holiday time, a family gathering, tax season, or vacation. Rather than starting on Monday, consider beginning on the weekend where there's often more temptation. That way you'll have more resolve and be on a routine when the weekend safely passes by and the week begins.

Get support. Tell your friends and family that you are serious about losing the weight that is making it harder for you to breathe. Ask for their support, not to nag you, but to encourage you, especially when they see you making good choices. It helps keep you on track when you've told others about your decision to lose weight.

If you have a friend or family member who is also trying to lose weight, you can have weekly weigh-ins and celebrate each other's victories, compare notes on what works, etc. You can also encourage E-mail friends to join your weight-loss program. Remember, however, that men tend to lose weight more quickly than women, so don't get discouraged if your buddy's a male and loses more weight faster than you do in the beginning.

If an informal friends' group doesn't work for you, consider joining a recognized weight loss program such as Weight Watchers or Take Off Pounds Sensibly (TOPS), or contact your local hospital to see if they have a program. Do not take pills "guaranteed" to help you lose weight. Many of them contain ingredients that can be harmful, especially if you have COPD.

Food substitutions. There are a number of lower-calorie substitutes that replace the higher-calorie foods you've been eating. For example, a dish of applesauce for a snack instead of a doughnut, skim milk instead of cream or even half and half, and whole wheat toast with jam instead of pancakes with syrup or a bagel with cream cheese. There are many good diet books listed in the "Suggested Reading" section of this book. But reading them won't help unless you make the effort to put what they have to say into practice.

Vary your diet. Variety is not only the spice of life, it's the best way to lose weight and still maintain the balanced diet you need to keep your respiratory muscles healthy, help reduce fatigue, and boost your immune system. Don't try fad diets or eat nothing but broccoli and sliced turkey.

Planning your weekly menus in advance can help you include variety. For example, rather than having half a cup of cereal every day for breakfast, occasionally eat a piece of whole wheat toast or half an English muffin with one ounce of low-fat cheese. One evening have three ounces of fish and the next night three ounces of chicken.

Think smaller. Many people who are overweight eat low-calorie foods, but they eat too much of them. Remember, three ounces is equal to the size of the palm of your hand (unless you have extremely large hands). Until you can begin to judge accurately, you might want to invest in a food scale, which is available at many groceries, pharmacies, kitchen equipment shops, and Weight Watchers.

Also, think smaller when it comes to your dinner plate. If you use a salad plate instead, your food will fill the space and it won't be as obvious that you have cut down on your portions.

Divide your plate. Experts suggest dividing your plate into quarters. Fill two of them with vegetables, one with protein (cheese, eggs, poultry, etc.), and one with grains such as brown rice, whole wheat bread, or barley.

Slow down. Eat more slowly. People who are overweight tend to chew their food less and gulp it down. Make a point to put down your spoon or fork between bites and not pick it up again until you've chewed carefully and swallowed what's in your mouth. Eating more slowly will help to reduce your shortness of breath because you'll have time to relax between bites.

Cut down on fat. Buy a small nonstick skillet so you can cook without adding fat. Otherwise, coat a regular skillet with a non-fat spray. Use a slow cooker or pressure cooker for roasts, stews, and stewed chicken. Then refrigerate the contents overnight. The fat will harden on top and you can scoop it off and throw it away. Many foods taste better the next day anyway as the seasonings have a chance to settle.

Don't cut out all fat. There's a tremendous difference in taste between low-fat cheese and no-fat cheese or low-fat mayonnaise and no-fat mayonnaise. If you don't like the way foods taste, you're not going to maintain a longtime commitment to losing weight.

Enjoy a free day. Give yourself one free day a week—not to gorge yourself but to let yourself enjoy that dish of ice cream or candy bar you've been craving. If you're too strict with yourself, those cravings will get stronger and you may go "off the wagon." Just don't declare a free day seven days a week.

Remember that you should try to lose only one to two pounds a week. It took a long time to gain the weight. Don't expect to lose it overnight.

When you've successfully reached the goal set by your physician, stop there and maintain that weight. The temptation is always to keep on losing just a little bit more. Don't do it. People with COPD who are underweight also have serious additional problems, so maintain the weight suggested by your physician.

EXERCISING

You may wonder how you can work exercise into your daily life since you find yourself breathless with almost all exertion. Yet proper exercise and techniques can help to keep you active, improve your self-confidence, improve your endurance, and help you to control and manage your breathlessness. Exercise can actually increase your respiratory capacity. That's why it's so important to attend your pulmonary rehabilitation classes and follow the directions of the nurses and other health care professionals who work with you in a safe environment.

■ Deconditioning Spiral

People with COPD often become frightened as they become more breathless, so they reduce their activity level in order to not have to struggle for air. But this action sets up a downward spiral in which you actually become less conditioned. As you reduce your exercise program, your muscle strength and your endurance decrease. Because your muscles become easily fatigued, they have to work harder to bring in air, and that, in turn, causes you to suffer from more breathlessness.

COPD affects your muscles as well as your lungs because of the lack of oxygen getting to those tissues. But as you exercise, you bring more blood with its oxygen into your muscles. The goal is to strengthen your muscles so they become more efficient and require less oxygen to do the same amount of work. You build endurance and improve your quality of life. It truly is a case of "use it or lose it."

■ What Types of Exercise Are Appropriate?

There is no one special exercise that is good for everyone. Your doctor will prescribe a particular exercise program designed expressly for you, taking into account your specific needs. But don't become a Sunday athlete, trying to get fit overnight. Take it slow as you go.

Progressive resistance exercise. Progressive resistance exercise uses large elastic exercise bands. By stretching these bands, you can improve upper-body strength and flexibility without suffering from too much shortness of breath (S.O.B.). This strengthening of your upper body is important for those many activities of daily living that require upper-body strength and flexibility, such as getting dishes down from a cupboard, taking a shower, making a bed, and even getting dressed.

Walking. One of the best exercises you can do, which your doctor will probably recommend, is walking. Begin slowly with a few steps and exhale using pursed-lips breathing. Then rest. Do this exercise five times a day.

Gradually increase your walking time to a minute without getting short of breath. Walk slowly around your house or, if the weather's good, outside to the mailbox and back. Then build up your endurance a minute at a time. Eventually, you'll be able to walk an hour without suffering extreme shortness of breath. But for now, just focus on the minute-by-minute progress. Keep a journal to show your improvement or mark the lengths of your walks on the calendar.

Even after you've built up energy and can walk half an hour or more, you need to warm up beforehand by walking slowly, then pick up your pace as is comfortable for you. You can use a tread-mill, especially in disagreeable weather (too hot, too cold, raining, or too windy) or if there is no safe place for you to walk. If you do have a safe place out-of-doors, however, walking in the fresh air and enjoying the beauty of nature can make exercise fun. Check first to be certain that the pollen count is not dangerously high and that the area in which you walk is reasonably free from air pollution.

Try to find a walking buddy. It makes sense for two reasons. First, you are more likely to walk if someone else is waiting for you and has scheduled that particular time for exercise. Second, it's a good idea in case you feel dizzy or breathless and need help finding a place to sit. Remember that the goal is endurance, not speed, and to walk without more than slight S.O.B.

Anytime you do feel out of breath, stop, relax, and do your pursed-lips breathing exercises. Then start again. While it's all right to push yourself a little, don't overdo. The idea is to build up your endurance, not to beat everyone around the block.

Swimming. Swimming is also a good exercise for those with access to a pool or lake, providing you stay close to shore and never swim alone. Water provides a buoyancy that makes you feel almost weightless and, as you probably remember from childhood, playing in the water is fun. However, if the chlorine chemicals in the pool trigger breathing problems, head for dry land.

Bike riding. Riding a bike—on a safe bike path or a stationary bike—strengthens your leg muscles and increases muscle tone and flexibility, which makes it easier for you to walk, climb stairs, and even dance. If you ride outdoors, stay away from roads with heavy traffic and gas fumes. L'Association Pulmonaire (the Lung Association) in Canada offers these suggestions when biking: "Control your breathing while exercising. Push the right pedal forward, breathe in, push the left pedal forward, and breathe out with pursed lips. Remember not to go too far, however, as you have to get yourself back. Ride to a secure location where you can stop and rest, if necessary before returning."

Bowling Many people with COPD are avid bowlers. Pick a ball that isn't too heavy and adjust your swing to your breathing. L'Association Pulmonaire offers these suggestions when bowling: "Don't rush. Take a deep breath, start breathing out with pursed lips and, at the same time, bend and bowl."

If there aren't any no-smoking bowling alleys in your area, learn when the slow times are and go bowling then.

Golf. If you can play golf without taking it too seriously, this can be a good source of fun and exercise. You can either walk slowly, pulling your clubs (along with your oxygen supplement, if needed), or ride in a cart.

Once again, L'Association Pulmonaire offers these tips when golfing: "Correlate your arm movements with your breathing pattern. Breathe in, position yourself, start breathing out with your pursed lips, and swing to hit the ball. If carts are permitted, you might want to take one in order to preserve your energy for hitting the ball. If carts are not permitted, take your time walking slowly. Rest when needed and let others play through."

Use your bronchodilator if necessary before teeing off. Even if you haven't played golf before, it might be fun to take some lessons.

Fishing. Fishing exposes you to fresh air, which boosts your appetite and helps you sleep like a baby. You get exercise casting your line, getting up to bait your hook and, of course, reeling in your catch. If you use supplemental oxygen, be sure to take enough with you if you go out fishing on a boat.

Take a friend or family member with you. It promises you hours to talk, share confidences, and maybe even to catch some fish. Some of my fondest childhood memories are fishing with my father and cherishing that special time alone with him.

Sailing. Sailing is another wonderful sport that combines exercise and fun. Be careful that it isn't too windy or, if it is, wrap a scarf around your mouth and nose so you don't inhale too much cold air.

There are numerous other activities, including gardening, and dancing, that you can do to keep your muscles active, even while using supplemental oxygen. Vary your activities so you don't become bored and quit exercising. You don't need to cut out many of the sports you enjoyed in the past, but you probably do need to make certain accommodations so you're more comfortable.

Just take your time, remember to use pursed-lips breathing, and have fun. That's what's life is all about.

Note: You must stop exercising immediately and notify your physician if you feel dizzy or experience nausea, muscle cramps, heavy sweating, or extreme breathlessness while exercising. Your physician may want to reevaluate your exercise plan from time to time.

The important point to remember is that you must continue to exercise unless your physician recommends against it. Bartolome R. Celli, M.D., of St. Elizabeth's Medical Center in Boston, notes in an editorial for the *American Journal of Respiratory and Critical Care Medicine* that studies worldwide have proved that pulmonary rehabilitation that includes exercise improves patients' outcomes. Exercise is better than any other form of therapy for increasing endurance and decreasing breathlessness in activities of daily living.

FAMILY AND FRIENDS

Coping with a friend or loved one who has breathing difficulties is a problem for many people. Some may begin to avoid social activities with you because they feel awkward and don't know what to say or how to act. Others, who still smoke, may see themselves reflected in your medical situation and don't want reminders of what may be lying ahead for them.

Your first impulse may be to write off these fair-weather friends. After all, you're the one who's ill. But if you do so, you're missing an important opportunity to educate others on COPD and show how a person can still have a rewarding life and enjoy a circle of support from others. Take time to make contact with a friend with whom you've lost touch. Tell him or her that you miss the friendship and specifically say how you'd like to renew it and also how the person can help you. Often, it isn't so much that friends don't want to be with you as that they feel helpless because they don't know what you need and don't know how they can help. Tell them.

■ If You Live Alone

If you live alone, you need to enlist the help of your friends in advance, just in case you begin to have serious breathing problems. Let them know what potential problems might arise. Ask one or more of them to call you each day just to make sure you're all right. (If you're going out or away on vacation, be sure to alert them, so they don't panic and call the paramedics.)

Keep a list of your medications and their doses, along with the name and phone number of your doctor, on the refrigerator, in case of an emergency.

If you live in an apartment or condo, get a siren or loud noise-maker that you can set off if you need to alert your neighbors that you need their help. Let them know about your alarm system ahead of time so they don't just write you off as a disruptive neighbor.

You can always call 911, even if you're having trouble talking because of a breathing problem. By staying on the line, the operator can trace your call and send an emergency team to you.

GETTING UP IN THE MORNING

Getting up in the morning can be a real problem for some people with COPD, especially if it's one of your "bad days" when you've had restless sleep and coughing spells that woke you when you did fall asleep. These hints might make things easier for you:

- If you have to be up at a specific time, rather than waking up abruptly to the noise of an alarm, set your clock radio to wake you to soothing music. There also are clocks that begin to glow when it's time to get up and progressively get brighter, which may be effective if you're a light sleeper in a dark room.
- Don't leap out of bed, even if you can. Instead, imitate a cat and try some gentle stretching and relaxation exercises before getting up. Then swing your feet over the edge of your bed. Wait a minute to catch your breath. Put your feet into your slippers (which you have left in easy reach) and slip on your robe. It will keep you warm if your room is on the cool side.
- If you prefer to dress before breakfast, put your shoes and socks by the bedside and your clothes either on the foot of the bed or on a chair or dresser right next to the bed at night before you retire. Invest in a long shoehorn (available in novelty shops, pharmacies, and some department stores) to help you slip into your shoes without bending over.

LIFTING AND CARRYING THINGS

Lifting heavy objects puts a strain on your heart and lungs, especially if, as most of us do, you tend to hold your breath as you lift.

- Whenever possible, avoid lifting. If you have to lift, breathe out as you bend at the knees, rest for a moment, then take a deep breath and exhale as you lift, holding the object close to your body to reduce strain. Practice this procedure and it soon will become second nature.

- Never carry things in your arms if you can push them or have someone else carry them for you.
- You can use a laundry basket with wheels for a myriad of other tasks such as holding your cleaning supplies, moving groceries from the car to your pantry or cupboard, and carrying your garbage to the trash cans outside or the trash chute if you live in an apartment.
- If you live in a two-story house, have a wheeled cart on both floors to keep you from having to carry things from room to room.
- If you have grandchildren who run to you and you want to swoop them up for a hug, sit in a chair instead and hug them without lifting them up.
- Ask for help if you need an item that's on a top shelf at the grocery or department store, especially if that item is heavy. If you're short, you may quickly realize that most of the smaller sizes are hung on the highest racks.
- At checkout, ask the person bagging your groceries to spread out the heavy items so the bags are lighter.
- Most supermarkets have people who will carry your groceries out to your car. Take advantage of this service.
- When you have to carry your own groceries inside, bring in the items that need refrigeration first, then rest before bringing in the nonperishables.
- If you're fortunate to live in an area where groceries are delivered, have yours delivered.

MAKING LOVE

Please note that this section is called "making love," not "having sex." This is done with intent because there is far more to making love than just having intercourse, and that's an important distinction for people with COPD and their partners.

The sex drive is a big part of a person's life, and that fact doesn't disappear when you have COPD. Yet for many COPD patients, sexual activity becomes a fond memory, often because the fear of breathlessness creates an overwhelming anxiety that just makes it easier to forget the whole thing.

Sexual functioning can be affected by COPD in a variety of ways. In a Spanish study of forty-nine patients, thirty-three had some type of sexual problem. First and foremost, the person with COPD must deal with shortness of breath and fatigue. In addition, many medications, as well as alcohol, can cause sexual dysfunction, including male impotence and a lack of desire for sex. Stress and depression, normal reactions to the diagnosis of COPD, can cause sexual dysfunction for both partners. The well partner's concern of "hurting" the loved one with COPD can also create barriers to lovemaking.

Unfortunately, many physicians and other health care professionals, due to their own embarrassment or ignorance with sexual issues, shy away from discussing sexual matters with their COPD patients or their partners. In addition, the myth that "older people don't do it" dies hard. Frequently, even medical professionals feed into that myth, by assuming that whoever is "old" by that particular doctor's standards is no longer interested in sex and so the subject doesn't need discussion. This omission leaves a couple depressed, embarrassed, frustrated, and fearful. If your physician seems uncomfortable answering your questions, consult a qualified sex therapist, marriage and family therapist, psychologist, or psychiatrist, or your minister, rabbi, or priest.

While there's no doubt that sexuality can be affected by COPD in a variety of ways, there are ways to compensate and bring lovemaking back into your life. Members of your support group may be able to share suggestions with you. It helps to know that they have faced the same problems you are facing and have discovered ways to compensate. Don't be reluctant or embarrassed to ask for help. There also is an excellent book on the topic of sexual relations, *Being Close*, that is available free from the National Jewish Medical Research Center by calling 1-800-222-LUNG.

■ Lovemaking Is Not Just Sexual Intercourse

It's often been said that the largest sex organ is between the ears. What this means is that our emotions often affect our interest and/or ability to enjoy sexual activity. For example, if a man's COPD has progressed to the point that he is no longer able to be the breadwinner and is dependent on his partner, he may feel "less manly" and a failure, and because of this, may suffer from impotency. A woman may feel less desirable if she needs to rely on oxygen. Both men and women may worry about breathlessness during sex or feel self-conscious about the use of oxygen.

Rather than just abandoning your sexual relationship, try to initiate open discussion about these problems with your partner. Discuss what is comfortable for both of you. Perhaps using Viagra to help stimulate an erection is an option. (Always check with your physician before taking any new medication.) Finding a time of day when fatigue is less of a concern is also important. Meanwhile, of course, there are other ways to maintain a close physical relationship, such as hugging, caressing, and old-fashioned necking, or by bathing or showering together. Intimacy is the goal, not necessarily intercourse and orgasm.

The Canadian Lung Association has created the following list of information by Susan King, an occupational therapist, to alleviate some of the anxiety around sexuality:

- COPD does not diminish sexual ability; it is only the frequency of sexual activity that is limited, as are all strenuous physical activities.
- The physical effort required for sexual intercourse is approximately equal to that required to climb one flight of stairs at a normal pace.
- Beginning an exercise program will help to build up the COPD person's tolerance to activity and in turn help to reduce shortness of breath with activity.
- Research findings show that the effort required for intercourse does not raise blood pressure, heart rate, and respiration to levels that are considered dangerous.
- Medication specific for your lungs will not affect your sex drive; however, if you are taking other medications (for example, antidepressants), it is important to ask your physician how these may interfere with your sex drive.
- Some changes in sexuality are not related to your lung disease but are normal changes with aging. For instance, slower erections and delayed orgasms are normal in middle and later life.

- Because of the physical effort required, it is important to have adequate rest both before and during sexual relations. In other words, plan your activity for your best time of day and rest at intervals during the activity if necessary.
- Clear bronchial secretions beforehand.
- Plan to have sexual activity immediately after using a bronchodilator.
- If you use supplemental oxygen for activity, plan to use the same amount of oxygen during sexual relations.
- Avoid sexual activity immediately after a heavy meal, after consuming alcohol, in an uncomfortable room temperature, or when under emotional stress. All of these factors increase your fatigability.
- Choose sex positions that are less energy consuming and that avoid pressure on the chest. For instance, the side-to-side position during intercourse is more comfortable and less tiring than the top-bottom position.
- Have the able-bodied partner assume a more active role so that the COPD partner doesn't become fatigued or anxious.
- Avoid allergic elements in the environment (perfumes, hair sprays) that may induce bronchospasm.
- Remember that simply touching, being touched, and being close to someone is essential to helping a person feel loved, special, and truly a partner in the relationship.

If you still have unanswered questions or concerns, be certain to ask your physician or other health care professional. This part of your life is too important to omit because of lack of communication. The American Association of Sex Therapists does not do counseling, but it can direct you to a certified sexuality counselor or therapist in your area.

American Association of Sex Therapists
PO Box 5488
Richmond, VA 23220-0488
AASECT@aasect.org

▨ Communication Gaps

Because human beings are essentially creatures of habit, some couples stop making love when the old way is no longer possible, rather than making adjustments, experimenting with other positions, or other foreplay techniques. The easy-breathing mate may feel as though he or she is taking advantage of the person with COPD and feel guilty for wanting sex, while the partner with COPD, who already may suffer from a loss of self-esteem, feels as though he or she is no longer sexually desirable. Usually, neither partner brings up the subject, creating even more distance between them at a time when both need reassurance and support.

Communication with your partner is the key to coping with not only sexual issues but also with all concerns of COPD.

MAKING THE BED

Beds probably create more problems than any other piece of furniture in the house. And it's not because of sexual problems, either. It's the great debate over making the bed.

For some, making the bed is a vital daily task that must be done because . . . well, just because. Others consider making the

bed to be a sign of being in control, of keeping things neat, of
starting the day right. But there are still others who have no
emotion connected to making the bed and if they don't get
around to it, they just pull the covers back and call it "airing the
bed."

Whether you have COPD or not, making the bed (especially
a king-size bed) can be tiring because it uses a great deal of
energy and requires strong upper-body movements. But if you
are in the "have to make the bed" school, you want to get the job
done. Here are a few tips that may make bed making easier and
less fatiguing for you:

- The easiest way to make your bed is to use a duvet, which
  is a blanket, often filled with down, encased in a sheet.
  Just slowly fluff up the pillows, inhaling as you raise your
  arms and exhaling through pursed lips as you drop the
  pillows on the bed. Then pull the duvet over the bottom
  sheet.
- Sit whenever you're tired.
- Try to get help when you change the bottom fitted sheet
  as it can be an exhausting task, especially if your bed is
  queen-size or king-size.
- If you don't use a duvet and prefer using a top sheet and
  blanket, try half making the bed while you're still in it.
  Pull the top sheet and blanket up on one side and
  smooth them out. Exit from the unmade side, which is
  then reasonably easy to finish.
- Remember that there's no law that you have to make
  your bed each day. Neatly fold the covers and top sheet

toward the foot of the bed and tell yourself (and others, if they need to know) that you're "airing" your bed.

PACING YOURSELF

You need to treat your energy level as a precious commodity, which it is. Take on only what you can handle comfortably and when you feel tired, QUIT. You're the only one who can honestly judge your energy level, so rule yourself wisely. Don't let others push you beyond your capacity and don't overexert yourself, trying to prove what a good sport you are.

There will, of course, be occasions when you want to push yourself a little because it would give you pleasure, such as going to a special niece's wedding, meeting a friend for lunch, or making love. It's all right to extend yourself a little if it's done with forethought and common sense.

- Wait until an hour or more after eating. Give your digestive system time to work, as digestion draws blood, with its oxygen, away from muscles, leaving them less able to cope with extra demands. This is why it's suggested that people wait an hour before exercising. Also, when your stomach is full it crowds your lungs, making breathing more difficult.
- You may find that you feel best soon after taking your medication or having a breathing treatment.
- If your physician has prescribed an aerosol inhaler, use it to help a special effort, but be careful to never use more than prescribed. More isn't always better and can be dangerous.

- Build in a "break time" during any activity where you may need to rest.
- Pace yourself and don't rush. It's better to plan ahead, even if it makes you arrive a little early to events. That way you can rest and catch your breath.
- If you feel breathless, use pursed-lips breathing (see Chapter 3). This really helps, so practice it so you feel comfortable using it anytime, anyplace.
- It's easier to pace yourself when you clear out unnecessary energy wasters such as retracing your steps, keeping possessions you no longer want or use, or continuing old habits that tire you out.
- Don't crowd your calendar. Many people find that they can handle only one activity per day, so don't plan on going out for lunch on the same day you have theater tickets, or go clothes shopping the same day you're having friends over for cards.

PLAYING

Although some of your previous recreational activities may be difficult to continue when your COPD progresses, you don't have to withdraw from contact with friends because you can't do what you used to do with them. There are many ways to enjoy each day, some in solitude, but many with friends.

First and foremost, says Francis W. Birch, who was diagnosed with emphysema two years after giving up smoking, "Be out and about. Join things. We joined a newcomers' group when we moved to the Cape and met some of the finest groups of friends. We even traveled with them."

Patricia Underwood, who was diagnosed with emphysema in January 2001, also remains an enthusiast for living. "I use liquid oxygen and never have to worry about losing power during storms," she said. "I also have a portable unit that allows me my freedom. I can't stress enough how important it is to keep on keeping on. The more you keep doing, the more you will be able to do. There is so much that I would like to say to encourage people. Too many people just sit inside and give up on the world. I have started wood carving and I am having a ball with it. Great gifts for Christmas, etc. We are going camping in September and I am pleased to go, hoses [from the oxygen tank] and all."

Other suggestions include:

- Join a COPD support group in your area. If there isn't one, talk to your local branch of the American Lung Association about starting one.
- Organize a regular group of friends to play mah-jongg, Scrabble, Monopoly, bridge, Boggle, or other games.
- Set up a permanent card table for jigsaw puzzles to be worked on alone or with family and friends.
- Hire a teenager from the local high school to teach you how to become computer literate.
- Trade books with friends so you always have something to read. Although you can get good books cheaply at flea markets and garage sales, be careful, as many of them are dusty and the pages may contain mold that might irritate your lungs.
- Write letters, that once popular art form, to distant friends and family. A letter is a permanent reminder that you're thinking of someone, which E-mail isn't.

- If you like chess, you can get computer chess games with varying levels of expertise, play through the mail with others, or over the Internet.
- If you want some quiet time for when you don't have much energy, do crossword puzzles. It exercises your brain as well.
- Join an adult education class at your local community college or university. If you don't have the energy for that, consider a correspondence course or take a class over the Internet.
- Learn a language with audio- or videotapes or with computer classes.
- Start a stamp or coin collection, needlepoint, or build scale models if your former hobbies create too much dust or take too much energy.
- Take piano or guitar lessons.
- Ask others about their activities. You might be surprised that some of their interests mirror yours.

RELAXATION TECHNIQUES

Both caregivers and those with COPD need to take time out for relaxation. Although naps are important because they can help reduce fatigue, specific relaxation techniques can help reduce stress and depression and offer peace of mind. These are not complicated exercises but proven techniques that can be done at any time during the day, whenever you feel the need. They'll help you to evoke what Herbert Benson, M.D., associate professor of medicine at Harvard Medical Institute and director of the Mind/Body Medical Institute, calls the "relaxation response."

"It's a calming state," says Benson in his book *Timeless Healing: The Power and Biology of Belief.* "The human body is geared to react by providing this calming state—the opposite of the fight-or-flight response—whenever the mind is focused for some time and disregards intrusive everyday thoughts. In other words, when the mind quiets down, the body follows suit."

These techniques include meditation, visualization, yoga, tai chi, progressive relaxation, music therapy, massage therapy, and self-hypnosis, just to mention a few. You don't need to do all of them, of course. Just try those that interest you most, and you'll soon find that you are able to relax yourself at will and reduce stress buildup without relying on medications. As 60 to 90 percent of all doctor visits in the United States are stress related, these relaxation skills should help reduce the number of times you need to see the doctor. While these techniques won't cure your COPD, they should help to make you feel better.

■ Avoid Energy Drainers (Human and Situational)

This is probably one of the most important things you can do to aid relaxation: Stay away as much as possible from people who drain your energy and who make you feel stressed. Just as most of us are drawn to individuals who have positive attitudes and face adversity with a smile, we are reluctant to spend much time with those who have a negative outlook, are "down" most of the time, and are constantly critical of others. Their negative feelings are catching. As the old song goes, "Accentuate the positive."

Even if, at first, you have to fake it, try being a little more upbeat. Look for what's good in life and in people. Before you know it, you won't be faking your positive outlook. It will have become an aspect of your being and you'll draw others to you because of it.

■ Exercise

It's important to realize the relaxation benefits of exercise, in addition to strengthening your muscles to help you breathe easier. Even when walking, you can focus on the rhythm of your steps, the sensations of the breeze against your face, the scent of flowers or fruit trees, or the sounds of birds, children laughing, or even cows mooing (and let's hope not of cars and trucks honking). The positive focus treats your various senses and wards against any thoughts that may cause you stress or concern. Some people repeat their mantra of "peace," "God," "love," etc., as they walk.

■ Humor

Although you may feel as though you have nothing to laugh about when you have COPD, most of the people I interviewed said laughter *was* the best medicine. Numerous studies have shown the benefits of laughter, describing how it relaxes muscles and stimulates the brain to release powerful chemicals called endorphins that help to reduce pain.

When you laugh you breathe deeply, bringing additional oxygen into your lungs. Laughing can reduce blood pressure and tension, and it improves blood circulation. It actually can stimulate your immune system by increasing the activity of T cells and so-called killer cells, keeping you healthier at a time when you need to be able to fight infection. It also can reduce depression, a natural response to COPD. Yes, laughing may trigger coughing and/or wheezing, especially if you have bronchitis or asthma, but overall, laughter makes you feel better. It also makes you look happier so others respond to you more positively (just as they tend to withdraw from those who look sad and unhappy).

Life does have its funny moments, and when you look for them and reflect on them, your spirits will lift. You've probably heard of the late Norman Cousins and his book *Anatomy of an Illness*, in which he described how laughter helped him to recover from ankylosing spondylitis, a painful and potentially crippling form of arthritis.

The importance of laughter is the theme of the World Laughter Tour, a group of health care professionals formed to help others improve their physical and mental health through systematic laughter. Founded in this country by psychologist Steven Wilson and Karyn Buxman, R.N., there are now more than one hundred clubs across the United States and Canada, where people meet to take part in "laughter exercise workouts and other activities that encourage playfulness, fun, and mental balance."

"It's important to dispel some myths about laughter," Wilson told me. "First, there is no medical evidence that anyone ever 'died laughing.' Second, humor is very personal. One individual may laugh at the antics of circus clowns while another laughs at Jay Leno jokes. What's important is that you laugh. Laughter's a physical art that's universal. Thirdly, you don't need a joke to laugh. Actually, only 10 percent of laughter comes from a joke while 90 percent of laughter is from social reasons. We laugh to look attractive, to show agreement, to feel pleasure.

"We're all born with an ability to laugh and smile," Wilson continued, "so even if you were raised in a serious family with an absence of laughter, I like to say it's never too late to have a happy childhood. But there's no doubt that many people suffer from 'sense of humor abuse.' We're taught not to laugh in church or in school. In our workshops, we encourage recollections of being criticized about laughter, that we laughed too loud, that we cackled, snorted, or were too silly. Our Laughter Clubs offer an environment where there's cheer, where people learn to laugh. We don't use racial, ethnic, or sexist humor. Our humor is uplifting and draws people together. Laughter helps people cope with their illness. Even an inner chuckle has good physiological benefits."

For more information about Laughter Clubs, call 1-800-669-5233 (614-855-4733 international) or go on-line at www.laughterclubs.com.

Although laughter can't cure COPD, it certainly can make you feel more upbeat as you live with it. You don't need to try to be a Jay Leno or a David Letterman. Just be yourself and you'll find humor in your own life.

Collect Humor

When you go to the video store, check out tapes and DVDs of movies that make you laugh. I've seen *Blazing Saddles* numerous times, but I still get a belly laugh from the slapstick humor. Your taste in humor may be more sophisticated, but there are hundreds of funny films to choose from. Post cartoons on your refrigerator and on your bathroom mirror. Buy joke books. Make it a point to see more of people who make you laugh and less of those who conduct ailing organ recitals when you get together.

Learn to Laugh at Yourself

Laughing at your own foibles makes you more human and gives others permission to laugh at themselves, too. It lifts the clouds of depression that are bound to follow you from time to time. If you look for humor in your life, you'll find it, often when you least expect it.

■ Journaling

For many people, writing in a journal or diary is a form of relaxation, especially when they focus on positive aspects of their lives—seeing friends, making love, traveling, or even daydreaming. According to some researchers, daydreaming, for many people, is analogous to relaxation and meditation, as it tends to relieve certain kinds of tension. And although writing a book such as this one is hard work at times, there certainly is a relaxing element to it, as it is almost impossible to think of other things when trying to "speak" to readers.

When you're writing in your journal, however, you write only for yourself. It doesn't matter if you're writing on the computer, in longhand in a composition notebook, or on a legal pad. You don't need a fancy journal for your writing. What you write is more important than what you write it in. Don't worry about spelling, punctuation, or vocabulary. You won't be graded.

The important aspect is to be honest. No one will read your

journal but you (unless you want others to). Explore your emotions, describe feelings, fears, and hopes. You're the expert in dealing with your disease, so write what's it's like for you.

Journaling can be cathartic. Having expressed your bad days in writing, you can move on to the good ones and may find, on reflection, that the good days are becoming more frequent, despite progressing symptoms, because you have learned to enjoy even the smallest joys in life.

Journaling often extends the emotional healing process to others as well because readers learn that someone else shares their fears, doubts, and frustrations. The late poet and author May Sarton published many of her journals. They not only were top sellers because they spoke to emotions others could relate to—fighting back from a stroke, aging, loneliness, and love of gardening—but they also served as a release for her.

■ Massage

For some, massage is the ultimate in relaxation; for others who don't enjoy being touched by strangers, it is a stressful event. For me, massage is a therapeutic necessity, not only aiding circulation but also working out the tension in my stress spots: my neck, shoulders, and forearms. Massage not only helps to reduce stress, but it also relieves symptoms associated with depression and insomnia, and helps to unlock breathing muscles stiffened from a chronic state of spasm. Massage reduces anxiety triggered by the struggle to catch a breath while it satisfies the human need to be a touched, a desire so strong that some infants who aren't stroked waste away.

According to Meryl Fury, a registered nurse at the Kenosha (Wisconsin) Community Health Center and a certified massage therapist, "The biggest benefit of massage in many ways is just being touched. People stop touching us as we get older, especially if we have a chronic illness because there's a fear of 'catching' it. For many seniors, their only human touch is an occasional kiss from the grandkids when they come to visit. Massage offers that human touch.

"Massage also increases circulation around the rib cage, most helpful to those patients with a barrel chest from struggling to breathe. It unlocks those muscles. There's also a strong mind/body connection in massage. People often have an emotional release. They'll cry or express sadness or anger. Most people with COPD," she added, "were dedicated smokers. They feel betrayed [by what cigarettes did to their lungs]. Massage often helps them to express those bottled up feelings."

Rebeccah Getz, an R.N. and certified massage therapist at the Martha Jefferson Hospital in Charlottesville, Virginia, is part of a program giving free massage to pulmonary and cardiac rehabilitation patients in the hospital. "We use a chair massage," she said, "and show the patients how to use massage to relax, especially the chest muscles used in breathing." Getz, a member of the American Massage Therapist Association, considers massage "a tool to prevent panic by using your body more effectively. It's not a cure for COPD, but it helps you deal with a chronic disease. You learn to work with your own body and have it work with you."

One of the exercises Getz has adapted for her COPD patients is the old nursery rhyme done by interlocking fingers, "Here is the church, here is the steeple. Open the doors and see all the people." The important aspect that helps breathing, according to Getz, is "interlocking your fingers as you curl your arms out with the thumbs down and elbows out." Then she has you pull your hands over your head to stretch, which opens the chest muscles.

There's nothing new about therapeutic massage. It was used as far back as the ancient Greeks and Romans and has been used by the Chinese, Japanese, and other Eastern cultures for centuries. Although there are different types of massage—Swedish, shiatsu, hot stone, sports massage, etc.—all involve some degree of stroking and kneading the body. They vary according to the amount of pressure applied and the type of stroke used.

Always check with your pulmonologist before arranging for a massage. If you have the okay, schedule your massage two or more hours after eating to avoid bloating and the risk of choking on regurgitated food. You also might want to use your inhaler a few minutes before a massage, just as you do before exercising. Remind your massage therapist to refrain from using scented oils or wearing perfume, as these scents may trigger coughing.

Many certified massage therapists, certified by your state, work in gyms, spas, and health clubs. You also can get referrals from an orthopedist or the physical therapy department of your local hospital or by contacting the American Massage Therapy Association, a professional organization of 46,000 members in thirty countries, at 1-888-843-2682 or on-line at www.amtamassage. org. The Web site gives you names and phone numbers of certified therapists in your area, and the type of massages they offer. You can request either a male or female massage therapist.

Although you need to remove your clothes before having a massage (unless it's a chair massage where the therapist is working only on your neck and shoulders), a sheet always covers your body. Some massage therapists will bring a table and come to your home. If you choose the latter, however, be sure to get references.

Always tell the massage therapist what type of massage you prefer—stroking, light feathery touch, deep work, etc. If you prefer no music in the background, say so. If the therapist is chatty, don't hesitate to ask him or her to stop talking so you can relax. Although I don't fall asleep during a massage as some people do, my mind usually goes blank for those sixty minutes, just taking in the warm sensation of my muscles being worked on and the state of relaxation.

Massages usually last thirty to sixty minutes, although Meryl Fury, a member of the American Massage Therapist Association, suggests that you might want to start with just fifteen. "Positioning is also important for those with COPD," she added. "Those individuals may not be able to lie on their back and will need pillows to support them and make them more comfortable." The cost for a massage is approximately $50 to $60 an hour. You'll probably pay more for a massage in a hotel or spa setting.

Even if you don't think you like to be touched, consider giving massage a try. You may like it and what it does for you.

■ Meditation

There's really nothing magical about meditation. To meditate, just find a quiet spot where you won't be interrupted, sit comfortably, and close your eyes. It helps me to picture a thick, black velvet curtain, with pile so thick you feel as though you could fall gently into it. Then find a word or words to repeat. It doesn't matter what you use. Some people prefer religious words such as "Jesus," "Lord," or "Allah." Others use "love," "peace," or "health," or a sound like "Ohmmmm."

Clear your mind of all other thoughts and just focus on your word or words as you slowly breathe in and out. As the mind can't hold two thoughts at the same time, unhappy or depressive thoughts will be crowded out as you focus on your word. Other thoughts will pop into your head at first, but just acknowledge them and let them float by like astronauts experiencing weightlessness and return to your focus on your breathing.

It's that simple: (1) focus on a meaningful word or phrase and (2) passively dismiss intruding thoughts and return to your focus on your breathing by murmuring your meaningful word or phrase.

As you evoke the relaxation response, your heartbeat and breathing slow down. Your muscles relax, requiring less blood flow to them. Your oxygen consumption actually decreases. Your body hangs up its fight-or-flight response and slips into something far more comfortable.

Dr. Herbert Benson suggests practicing this technique for ten to twenty minutes once or twice a day. Don't worry about the results. There's no competition and no prizes to be handed out. Be patient if it takes you a while to learn to relax. You wouldn't expect to become an expert golfer or piano player the first day out. Just keep trying and you'll get the hang of it. Remember the success of the tortoise.

Stress-reduction techniques are a lot like the waterproofing chemical the dry cleaners put on your raincoat after it's been cleaned. If they don't add this protective coating to make it waterproof again, your coat will absorb water like any other non-waterproof garment. Similarly, stress-reduction techniques won't eliminate stress from happening in your life any more than a waterproofed raincoat eliminates rain. But both can protect you from getting soaked.

■ Music Therapy

In 1697, English playwright William Congreve wrote, "Music hath charms to soothe a savage breast, To soften rocks, or bend a knotted oak." Music has far more than charms, however. It also possesses great therapeutic powers.

Music therapy is hardly a modern concept. The Bible tells of King David, who played on his harp to cure Saul of his depression. Ancient physicians used singing and crude musical instruments to bring a rapid heartbeat under control and to otherwise comfort their patients.

Doctors today are once again learning to accept music therapy as a powerful way to treat pain and anxiety. Dr. Mathew Lee, director of the Rusk Institute of Rehabilitation Medicine, New York University Medical Center, stated at a government hearing in August 1991, "Music therapy has been an invaluable tool with many of our rehabilitation patients. There is no question that the relationship of music and medicine will blossom because of the advent of previously unavailable techniques that can now show the effects of music."

According to the American Music Therapy Association (AMTA), there are about five thousand practicing music therapists in the United States on staff in hospitals, or working in outpatient clinics, rehabilitation facilities, and other venues. Board certified music therapists use music to promote movement with physical rehabilitation, as well as to alleviate pain in conjunction with anesthesia or pain medication, elevate patients'

mood and counteract depression, calm or sedate, often to induce
sleep, counteract apprehension or fear, and lessen muscle tension
for the purpose of relaxation. For more information about music
therapy, contact AMTA at 301-589-3300 or visit their Web site
at www.musictherapy.org.

You can use music to help you relax on your own as well. Sitting quietly with your eyes closed, listening to soothing music,
helps to relax tension in your body, which, in turn, triggers the
release of endorphins, the body's natural painkillers. Endorphins
reduce your brain's perception of stress and can create positive
changes in your mood and emotional state.

Experiment with different types of music to discover what
works best for you. If you listen to a classical music station on
the radio, choose one that is free from continual commercial
interruptions.

■ Progressive Relaxation

Progressive relaxation is relearning to relax your muscles,
something you knew how to do as a baby. As an infant or toddler, you let your body go limp whenever and wherever you were.
You were able to go to sleep in the car, at the table, on your par-
ent's shoulder, or on the floor. The theory is that if you are
relaxed, you cannot be tense.

To relearn this habit, lie down and close your eyes. Focus on
each part of your body, beginning with your forehead. Exhale
and tell yourself to relax your forehead and enjoy the sensation
as those muscles obey. Then move to your cheeks, your mouth,
your neck, and work down your body until you get to your toes.
Exhale gently as you focus on each body part. With each pro-

gressive step, take time to enjoy the sense of relaxation you feel in that muscle group. With your mind focused on that, the thoughts of stress you may be experiencing in the real world are locked out. Visualize those problems or extraneous thoughts actually moving away from you as though you were a magnet and had reversed the magnetic field, thus repelling all stressful thoughts and forming a safe protective barrier around yourself.

Practice progressive relaxation once or twice a day for ten to twenty minutes, but no more than that. "The idea is not to withdraw from the world," a psychologist told me, "but to be equipped to handle stressful situations by being able to relax and release the tension you feel."

■ Tai Chi and Yoga

Yoga and tai chi are two ancient forms of relaxation that aid the body by focusing the mind. Both exercise techniques combine specific breathing patterns, postures, and focused attention. Tai chi consists of slow, meditative motions and is especially helpful in improving balance, strength, and range of motion. Yoga gently stretches and relaxes the muscles.

You can get videotapes demonstrating yoga and tai chi, even some with the instructor facing away from you so you don't get confused on which arm or leg to use. However, I think it's easier to learn the basics by working with a live instructor who can correct your stance and show you firsthand how to do certain positions. Most community centers and some hospital wellness centers offer classes in both yoga and tai chi. Be sure to check with your physician before signing up for either of these classes.

▪ Visualization

Visualization is very similar to meditation, except that instead of focusing on a word or phrase, you try to re-create in your mind a physical scene that makes you feel at peace with the world. It can be a favored location from childhood, a place where you felt happiest, or a relaxing vista seen only in your imagination. For some, it may be merely lying in a hammock, feeling the warmth of the sun, hearing birds chirping, and experiencing the slow back-and-forth movement as the breeze makes the hammock sway. Use all your senses as you experience this place of comfort.

Begin by getting comfortable, closing your eyes, and taking as deep a breath as you can. Repeat twice more. Then allow your mind to carry you to a perfect place you find beautiful, a scene that fills you with a sense of calm, your "safe haven."

My visualized "safe place" is an old-fashioned rope swing that sits on top of a hill. It overlooks a harbor filled with large sailing ships. I let myself taste the salt air and feel the breeze against my cheeks as I swing back and forth. I've decided that the motion of the swing takes me back to the days of my childhood, when there was no sense of urgency and few responsibilities, when I could swing for hours watching a butterfly fluttering over a flower or finding animal forms in the clouds overhead. This specific scene fills me with a sense of peace and calmness, and I often revisit it when I feel a need to unwind.

As with meditation, thoughts of today's concerns may pop in, causing your mind to wander from time to time. Let them pass and return to your visualized special place. With practice, you'll find visualization an easy way to relax when you begin to feel stressed.

You also can use visualization to picture in your mind what

you'd like to achieve, a process known as goal imagery. Athletes often use visualization to see themselves making free throws, hitting a golf ball, running faster, or performing a perfect dive. Studies throughout the world show that athletes who visualize themselves performing their sport, step by step, actually move the muscles needed to perform that action, creating a mental blueprint for when they do it "for real." Actors use visualization to help them create a particular role, and public speakers use visualization to see themselves connecting positively with their audience. As Bernie Zilbergeld, Ph.D., and Arnold A. Lazarus, Ph.D., say in their book *Mind Power: Getting What You Want Through Mental Training*, "When you regularly imagine having achieved your goal, you are changing who you are."

Obviously, visualizing yourself without COPD isn't going to cure your disease and make you a marathon runner. But you can visualize yourself achieving the goal of walking a longer distance without getting breathless or enjoying your family, free of fatigue. Don't doubt the power of visualization. Actor Christopher Reeve has and is using visualization along with other techniques to fight his paralysis. He is now able to move his fingers and is regaining tactile feeling throughout his body, to his doctors' amazement. As Walt Disney said, "If you can dream it, you can do it."

So see yourself exercising in order to have less breathlessness. Visualize yourself enjoying sports and social activities without falling out with fatigue. Make your visualizations as real as you can by using all your senses. Visualize the results you want and see yourself carrying out the actions necessary to achieve them. Visualization works.

RESTING

Frequent rest times are important to reduce fatigue and help your breathing. If you don't have one of those wonderful chaise longues that movie stars of old were often seeing relaxing in, opt for a comfy couch, a chair with a footstool, or your bed. Sometimes just ten minutes to half an hour will make you feel better.

When you're resting, try to eliminate distractions by letting your answering machine pick up your phone when it rings, closing the window if the lawn mower motor is too loud or the neighborhood kids are playing and shouting. Allow your mind to clear itself. It just takes a little time, like when you stir up water in a fish tank and then watch it settle. Relax, close your eyes, and enjoy your rest. Before you know it, you'll have energy again for playing.

SHAVING

- It's less fatiguing to sit down as you shave. If you have a mirror that swings on a hinge, you can position it so you can see yourself even from a sitting position.
- Put all of your shaving gear on a tray near to the sink where you shave. That will save unnecessary steps.
- Many men and women prefer shaving with electric razors, claiming they require less physical energy to use. Try it if you find using a razor and shaving cream too tiring.
- Avoid shaving cream and after-shave lotions that contain perfume. They can irritate your lungs and make you cough or gasp for breath.

SHOPPING

Shopping is usually divided into two groupings: that which you have to do (grocery shopping) and fun shopping (shoes, etc.). Both types, however, expend a great deal of energy and so require you to plan ahead.

- Use lists for grocery shopping, errands, and even fun shopping. A list helps you remember what you need, and allows you to plan your trip so you don't waste time and energy having to double back to where you have been. Ask family members to write down needed items (toothpaste, toilet paper, stamps, etc.). If it's not on the list, you don't buy it.
- Shop when the stores aren't busy. Usually, that's early in the morning. Grocery stores are often busiest on Thursday and Friday afternoons and on weekends. Stores, especially in malls, tend to be most crowded on weekends.
- Use a shopping cart or an electric cart, if the grocery has them, and ask someone to help you with heavy items or those on shelves over your head.
- Ask the bag person to put your perishable items in a separate bag so you can just unload those if you are too tired to bring in everything.
- If you have to haul your groceries inside the house by yourself, ask the bag person to load the bags only half full.
- Also accept the bag person's offer to help carry your bags out and load your packages in your car. Have them put in the trunk because it's easier to lift bags out of the trunk

than from the backseat of the car, especially if you have a two-door car.

- Rest between carrying in grocery bags.
- For clothing and other items, shop on-line or through catalogs whenever possible. Trying on clothes is exhausting for most of us, so if you're too tired to try things on, ask to have them on approval, with the understanding that you can return them if they don't fit.
- If you feel you must try on clothes before buying, wear a shirt that buttons, rather than having to pull it over your head, and shoes that slip on. It makes it easier to get undressed and dressed without becoming too tired.
- Always wash your hands when you get home from shopping. Bacteria lingers on doorknobs, grocery cart handles, and other surfaces you might have touched. I always carry a few antibacterial hand wash packets in my purse. Be sure to buy only those that are unscented.

TRAVEL

Don't let COPD clip your wings if you have travel fever. You can still travel; it just takes some advance planning. Wherever you travel, whether to downtown or Down Under, there are some general suggestions to consider.

- Discuss your travel plans ahead of time with your physician.
- Avoid traveling during rush hours or holiday time, if possible. Not only are there too many crowds to deal

with, you also won't get the attention and service you
may need from those in charge.

- Buy tickets and reserve seats ahead of time so you don't
  have to stand in line.
- Minimize your luggage. Use suitcases on wheels, but
  check what you can and carry on only a small bag of
  necessities such as medications.
- Always carry your medicines with you. Never put them
  in checked luggage.
- Be prepared, as the Boy Scouts say, in case you develop a
  respiratory infection while you're away. Carry an antibiotic with you along with your physician's written instructions on how and when to increase your bronchodilator
  dosage.
- Remember that "mile-high" cities such as Denver, Salt
  Lake City, and Mexico City not only tend to have less
  oxygen in the air but also may have high levels of air pollution. Check with your physician if your travel plans
  include cities such as these.
- If you require time-determined medications or oxygen,
  be sure you have an adequate supply if there are delays or
  surprise cancelations.
- Always get travel insurance in case you need to cancel or
  postpone your trip because of illness.
- Carry a letter from your doctor, saying why you need
  supplemental oxygen, in case you are stopped by security.
- Plan ahead to give yourself plenty of time to get to your
  destination, so you don't feel anxious or experience additional stress.

■ **By Car**

- If you're driving or being driven in someone's car, be sure there's no scent of perfume or cigarette smoke in the upholstery.

- You're better off not driving at all when there's an ozone alert in your area. Polluted air from outside can be drawn into your car through the fan.

- Ask your doctor to write a letter to the Division of Motor Vehicle Registration authorizing you to get a handicap-parking sticker. This permit will let you park closer to stores so you don't have to walk so far. Don't let pride keep you from benefiting from this important perk. It was created for people who have physical health problems, and you certainly qualify. Save your energy for the shopping.

- If the price isn't too much more than self-service, use the full-service area when you need to fill the car with gas so you can avoid inhaling the fumes. If you need to do the pumping, stand upwind from the pump to prevent gas from spilling on you or your inhaling the fumes as they swirl by.

- If you get your car washed at a commercial car wash, warn the attendants not to automatically squirt "air freshener" inside the car. It will take days for the scent to dissipate, and meanwhile, the odor can trigger coughing.

- Always carry a cell phone with you, in case there's an emergency. For safety's sake (and in some states, to obey the law), pull off the road before you use it.

■ **Public Transportation**
  • If you're not driving a car (or being driven), most COPD experts (those individuals with the disease) suggest not traveling by subway if possible. The staircases are too steep with too many steps to climb, the air quality is poor, and people tend to push to get on or off. Often people are wedged in tightly like the proverbial sardines, subjecting you to their coughing, sneezing, perfume fumes, and remnants of cigarette and cigar smoke.
  • Take a bus or taxi instead, as smoking is no longer permitted in these vehicles. If you use a public bus, try to ride during off hours when it isn't so crowded and sit toward the front so you don't inhale the fumes from the exhaust.

■ **By Air**

Air travel is obviously the fastest way to get from destination A to destination B, providing there are no delays so you miss a connecting flight or your flight isn't canceled.

Jo-Von Tucker, who has had COPD for fifteen years and is dependent on supplemental oxygen use 24/7, nevertheless travels a great deal. She urges those who are also on oxygen and are thinking about flying to plan ahead. You're not permitted to bring your own portable oxygen unit on board and need to notify your airline of your plans about two weeks in advance.

Jo-Von admits that, since September 11, flying has become more difficult for those who are dependent on supplemental oxygen. She reports, "I've noticed much tighter security, even in a wheelchair and with oxygen. Have had to remove my shoes, etc. Stand up for pat-down searches. Explanations to unknowledgeable security people about supplemental oxygen and equipment. Longer times must be allowed for check-in. But, in general, most airline personnel have been very good.

"Additional arrangements are necessary for getting an escort through security to bring my portable oxygen tank back from the gate after my departure. A pass must be issued to that person at the ticket counter. Take extra copies of your oxygen prescription with you, as they will be needed (and possibly must be left with the various ticket agents, etc.). Cost of oxygen on board has gone up to $75 per flight segment. A trip to Kansas City is costing me $300 for oxygen on the plane, more than the cost of my ticket. Then I have to pay the oxygen company at the destination $100 to meet me with a filled portable at baggage claim. And O_2 must be set up for me at the hotel where I'm staying. Another $300+. Figure it out yourself. The cost of traveling with supplemental oxygen is pretty much prohibitive for most COPD patients."

- Most airlines have a medical department, and you should contact it to learn its unique requirements. You can also check your carrier's Web site. United, for example, requires forty-eight hours' advance notification and a list of medical information including passenger's name and age along with physician's name and contact information (with office hours). They also require a diagnosis from the physician. Although you must use equipment provided by United, they will transport your equipment providing it meets their packaging and labeling requirements.
- Whenever you travel by air, request a wheelchair to take you to the plane and meet you when you arrive at your

destination. It saves the energy you'd use walking from terminal to terminal for more enjoyable activities and allows you to board early so you can get yourself and your equipment settled before the hordes pour into the aisles.

Trains

The advantage of train travel is that you can take your portable oxygen with you, although you need to give advance notice. The disadvantage is that you can't stop along the way when you need to refill and, for that reason, experts suggest that you carry a safety margin of 20 percent. Although the upholstery in the seats may be dusty, train travel is a pleasant and relaxing way to travel short distances. For more information, contact Amtrak at 1-800-872-7245.

Cruises

Many people with COPD prefer to vacation on cruise ships. They like the sense of security provided by knowing there's a ship's doctor on board while enjoying the fresh air and variety of programs provided for passengers. If they tire, their room is nearby. You don't have to stray far from home either, as many itineraries hug the coast of North America. Some, like paddlewheel ships, cruise up and down the Mississippi, a real treat if you've never seen just how wide that river is.

If cruising appeals to you, check well in advance with the particular line to see if they permit passengers with supplemental oxygen to travel with them and what their specific requirements are, as each cruise line is different.

Carnival Cruise Lines, for example, requires a letter from your physician saying it is safe for you to travel, along with the type of oxygen you'll be using and the container. They stress that you need to bring enough for the entire cruise as they cannot furnish extra if you run out. For additional information, contact Carnival's Special Access at 1-800-438-6744, extension 70025.

Crystal Cruises has a more formal specification list, requiring those using supplemental oxygen to sign a release and indemnity from holding Crystal Cruises harmless and agreeing to the stipulations outlined, which are summarized below:

1. You must provide a letter from your physician stating that you require oxygen for your medical condition and are fit to travel and for the specific cruise, and that provides the prescribed oxygen flow (liters/minute).

2. You must travel with a companion who knows how to use your oxygen equipment.

3. You must make all arrangements for (and pay for) an oxygen concentrator and portable compressed gas oxygen equipment to be delivered to the ship before sailing and to be picked up from the ship at the end of the cruise. You must supply information about the supplier and equipment at least fourteen days before the sailing date.

4. Only oxygen concentrators and portable compressed gas cylinders are allowed. Liquid oxygen equipment is not allowed. Portable bottles are limited to not larger than cylinder size "E" (36 inches long).

5. If the oxygen equipment is not delivered to the ship in time for sailing, you and your companion will not be allowed to sail.

6. Crystal's ships are capable of providing only limited medical services. In the event your equipment malfunc-

tions or you develop medical complications, you and
your companion may be required to disembark and
return home at your own expense.

7. The number of oxygen-dependent guests is limited to
   two for any cruise because of limited storage for oxygen
   cylinders.

8. You can travel only on those cruises on which you can
   be properly supported by equipment vendors and that
   have itineraries that will easily allow medical disem-
   barkation if you need it. This includes only cruises that
   begin and end in a U.S. or Canadian port.

As you can see, supplemental oxygen requirements are very
cruise-specific, so be sure to check with the particular cruise line
you plan to use.

■ International Travel

Although many individuals with COPD travel internationally
without difficulty, be warned that you'll find smokers everywhere,
especially in France, Spain, Italy, and Ireland. Although some
restaurants in Great Britain and on the Continent have no-
smoking sections, you'll find secondhand smoke wafting on the
streets, in hotel lobbies, and in most restaurants. Keep that in mind.

What's more, you need to be careful when you make reserva-
tions at centuries-old picturesque châteaus or castles. Their
charm, of course, is that they are old, but with age comes centuries of mold and dust. I developed a respiratory infection in
one of France's best from breathing in dust and mold from the
heavy velvet curtains that surrounded the bed and probably
hadn't been cleaned in years, if ever. Also think twice about

lighting the romantic fireplace in your room. The smoke and ash may affect your breathing as well as your passion.

Don't let the need for advance planning cause you to throw up your hands and decide to stay home. Well-planned traveling can be enjoyable, stimulating, and educational. It provides a needed change of pace and wonderful memories and may remind you that there's more you can do than cannot.

For additional information concerning traveling, you can contact the Society for Accessible Travel & Hospitality (SATH), formerly the Society for the Advancement of Travel for the Handicapped, which was founded in 1976. SATH is a nonprofit educational organization offering worldwide listings of accessible facilities including flights, cruises, vans, hotels, and tourist attractions.

347 Fifth Avenue, Suite 610
New York, NY 10016-4010
Tel: 212-447-7284
Fax: 212-725-8253
sathtravel@aol.com
www.sath.org

UNDRESSING

Sit on your bed or on a chair when you get undressed. Kick off your shoes first. Then slip out of your slacks or skirt. Rest a few minutes before unbuttoning your blouse or shirt and removing your socks. Then rest again before getting into your nightclothes. Undressing is often more difficult than dressing in the morning because you're more fatigued. Take your time.

VOLUNTEERING

You may think it odd that I include volunteering as an activity of daily living, but I think that the simple act of volunteering makes our lives worth living. In giving of yourself, you receive much more in return. It boosts your sense of self-worth, leaves a little of you in the lives of those you've helped, and just makes you feel good, especially when you reach out to young people.

My good friend, author, educator, and psychologist Sol Gordon, writes of "Mitzvah therapy" in his book, *When Living Hurts*. According to Gordon, "I only know of two ways to promote self-esteem in young people. One of them is to teach them a new skill so that they have a sense of achievement, a pride in something they can do. The other is to get youngsters who feel miserable about themselves to do good deeds—mitzvahs—to be helpful to those in need of a helping hand."

Think about it. What skills do you have that you can share with others, especially young people who need to feel more cared for, more capable, and more communicative? Can you knit or cross-stitch, whittle or make model airplanes? Write poetry, do bookkeeping, or draw? Do you know about first aid, cooking, or storytelling? Share your talent with a young person in the Boy Scouts or Girl Scouts, Boys and Girls Club, Police Athletic League, or a church or synagogue group. It will give you a sense of purpose if you're no longer able to work, a sense of joy to see how the youngsters respond to your attention, and a sense of confidence that you're educating our country's future citizens about the dangers of cigarette smoking, the importance of giving back to others, and intergenerational communication.

There are other ways you can give something back to your

community. Are you a former teacher? If so, get in touch with a local school and offer to help tutor children in reading or math, teach English as a second language to our newest citizens and citizens-to-be, or teach a contemporary to read.

Are you a retired business executive? There are many fledging businesses who could benefit from your expertise. If you were a professional health care worker, offer your volunteer services at our many non-profit health organizations who would really welcome your help.

Even if you've never been gainfully employed, you probably have experience in organizing events, running your church or synagogue committees, or giving parties. If you don't have the energy to do those activities today, you still can share your wealth of information with others and be proud of the contribution you've made. Remember, the word "volunteer" has a "U" in it.

WORKING

Once you've been diagnosed with COPD, many thoughts may whirl through your mind, some of which focus on how long you can keep on working. Obviously, a good portion of the decision rests on the nature of your present job. If you're a teacher, commercial fisherman, or carpenter, for example, you may find that eventually the physical energy required for you to do your job properly is just too much. On the other hand, occupations requiring less physical energy, such as bookkeeping, writing, selling, dressmaking, and consulting, may be continued even if you're on supplemental oxygen.

■ Meet with a Vocational Counselor

Talk to a vocational rehabilitation counselor to learn if it's possible, with modifications, to continue your present occupation and, if not, how you can adapt your talents and interests into a new endeavor that allows you to go back to work even with the limitations COPD has placed on you. Your counselor will evaluate your potential through interviews, pulmonary function and exercise stress tests, and standard interest questionnaires.

If you're in a pulmonary rehabilitation program, there should be a vocational rehabilitation counselor working with you. If not, check your local phone book for the number of the Department (or Division) of Rehabilitation or Rehabilitation Services. If you have access to a computer and modem, try the National Clearinghouse of Rehabilitation Training Materials Web site at www.nchrtm.okstate.edu/index_3.html or call their toll-free number, 1-800-223-5219.

■ Retrain for the "New You"

Don't just throw in the towel and picture yourself as completely physically disabled. There may be new occupations, even on a part-time basis, where you can continue to be productive, feel (and be) needed, and earn extra income. If you're artistically inclined, think about painting vases and trays to be sold along with knitting or needlepoint items in a gift shop. Take art lessons and you may discover an unexpected talent. (Grandma Moses was seventy-six when she started painting.) You're never too old to write a book. If you're gifted in math, offer to tutor some youngsters. Bilingual? Give Spanish or French lessons. It isn't just keeping you busy, you know. It's keeping your mind active as well.

You may need to rethink your self-identity. We often tend to think of ourselves in terms of our work—"I'm a doctor" or "I'm a decorator," rather than who we are as a person (a man or woman, a mother or father, husband or wife, happy individual, loving and caring human being). If you've been defining yourself by your profession, career, or job, it may be more difficult to alter your thinking if you can no longer carry on that particular occupation. If you're struggling with a sense of a loss of identity, talk to a professional counselor.

Although many people with COPD find that they eventually are not able to continue their full-time job, it doesn't mean you should stay home watching television. There are many part-time jobs available that can provide extra money and at the same time give you the opportunity to meet other people and continue to feel useful. Watch the want ads in your paper and tell everyone you know that you're looking for work. That's how most people find their jobs.

Perhaps you can become a consultant in the field in which you used to work. Many businesses, especially small businesses, hire consultants when needed from time to time. If you're knowledgeable about bookkeeping, you could keep books for a non-profit agency or a small business. I had a friend who prepared taxes for a number of people for many years. She made enough income out of her "little business," as she called it, that she and her husband were able to enjoy many trips to Europe.

If you're handy, you can do minor repairs or paint, do needlework, or make crafts to sell during the holidays and at the many craft bazaars that crop up in all communities. For those who are computer whizzes, your list of potential clients will be endless. In my community, a high school student had so many clients needing help with their computer problems that he had to hire helpers (also high school students).

The important message here is that there is too much to do, and too much good to do in the world and in your community, for you to sit idle if you feel well enough to work. Roll up your sleeves, use your imagination, and put your talents to good use. Antoinette Brown Blackwell, feminist, writer, and first ordained woman minister in the United States, who lived from 1825 to 1921, phrased it perfectly when she wrote, "Work, alternated with needful rest, is the salvation of man or woman."

Yes, there are a multitude of changes that enter your life when you're diagnosed with COPD, but change is a normal part of the human condition. It's how we adapt to change that makes the difference. My grandmother used to say, "Anyone can do just fine when all's going right; it's how you behave when problems arise that shows your mettle as a person." Throughout my life, I've discovered that Grandmother was right.

6

Conclusion

Although at present, there is no cure for COPD, there are ways to slow the progression of the disease and to help you live a more fulfilling life. So don't give up hope.

Researchers are working on a number of drugs that, if successful, can ease the burden of those suffering from the symptoms of COPD.

- Longer-acting bronchodilators, which may require only one daily dose, are currently in clinical trials and may be available shortly.
- Scientists are working to discover new drugs that can lessen the body's natural rejection for those undergoing lung transplants without making you, as the recipient, susceptible to infection.
- Studies on new anti-inflammatory drugs for COPD are currently underway.

Future hopes include:

- More genetic studies on COPD to predetermine which individuals are more susceptible to COPD.
- Better ways to predict which patients might benefit from lung volume reduction surgery.
- Better and safer ways to conduct lung volume reduction surgery.
- Xenotransplantation (transplanting organs from animals for use in humans). Research is being done on the development of transgenic pigs as their physiology is similar to humans and their organs are about the same size. Just as pig heart valves are now being used on humans, perhaps pig lungs could be used as well, making the supply of available lungs far greater and shortening the waiting time to find a suitable donor.
- The creation of a treatment that can trigger the destroyed alveoli to regenerate new and healthy tissue. "After all," says Richard Casaburi, Ph.D., M.D., "other body parts can be regrown to some extent, even in adults (fingernails, skin, etc.)."
- New drugs that can control the pulmonary inflammation and destruction of tissues that occurs in COPD.
- New technologies to create more efficient and compact supplemental oxygen delivery systems to help people remain active even while on supplemental oxygen.

This is not all just wistful thinking. Work is being done throughout the world to find better ways to increase awareness of COPD and to prevent, diagnose, and treat this disease. The Global Initiative for Chronic Obstructive Lung Disease

(GOLD) is a collaborative project of the World Health Organization and the National Heart, Lung, and Blood Institute, developed to unify international efforts in the management of COPD.

Peter Calverley, M.D., a physician at Fazakerley Hospital in Liverpool, England, is a member of GOLD's executive and dissemination committees. "Hopefully, the future for COPD sufferers will be brighter than the past," he said. "Earlier diagnosis, using objective criteria, should allow informed treatment decisions to be made. New research into the mechanisms producing this disorder will generate novel approaches to disease management that will reduce the burden of COPD."

Another group working on answers to the questions of COPD prevention, diagnosis, and management, is the Pulmonary Education and Research Foundation (PERF). Richard Casaburi, Ph.D., M.D., and president of PERF, offered his ideas on some changes this century will bring to the prevention, treatment, and hopefully, cure for COPD.

"There is a growing perception that, if we try really hard, we can make progress in finding new therapies for COPD. The concept that the airway obstruction is totally irreversible is being challenged. Best of all, there are starting to be hints that powerful new medical sciences may someday discover ways to repair lungs that until now we have thought of as irredeemably destroyed.

"Rehabilitation is emerging as the technique of choice to improve the function of everything *except* the lung. It has been discovered that it is not only the lung that functions poorly in the COPD patient. For example, psychological dysfunction (depression) often keeps a patient homebound and isolated. Psychosocial interventions that are part of pulmonary rehabilitation make the patient more functional and improve quality of life. Therapies that improve muscle function have been shown to improve exercise tolerance. This is of tremendous importance as it has been argued that exercise training is more effective than either bronchodilators or oxygen therapy in decreasing the shortness of breath that occurs in everyday activities, thus improving the patient's quality of life."

So, even though you struggle with some of the effects of COPD, don't give up hope for new drugs, new therapies, and hopefully, a cure for COPD. Continue to live your life to the fullest, enjoying the riches of family, good friends, good food, interesting travel, and the myriad pleasures that make life worth living. If you need medications and supplemental oxygen to make all that possible, so be it. My wise grandmother often said, "Everybody has something. This is what you have." She wasn't being abrupt. She was stating reality.

You can choose to hide away in your home, waiting for the end to come, or you can determine to make the most of every day. The choice is yours. America's first first lady, Martha Washington, believed that, saying "The greater part of our happiness or misery depends on our dispositions and not our circumstances."

In *Enjoying Life with Chronic Obstructive Pulmonary Disease*, perhaps authors Thomas L. Petty and Louise M. Nett summed it up best: "Somehow, the human spirit possesses an ability to adapt and grow, which we believe can be awakened and kindled for the pursuit of happiness at any time in life."

Good luck and God bless.

Resources

General Resources

Alpha1 Association
8120 Penn Avenue South, Suite 549
Minneapolis, MN 55431-1326
1-800-521-3025 or 612-703-9979
fax 612-703-9977

AINA@alpha1.org
www.alpha1.org
815 Connecticut Ave NW
Suite 1200
Washington, DC
20006-4004
202-887-1900
800-521-3025
A nonprofit organization that
provides support, information, and
reading material for those with the
genetic susceptibility for COPD and
their families.

American Association for
Respiratory Care
11030 Ables Lane
Dallas, TX 75229

972-243-2272
www.aarc.org

American Association of Sex
Therapists
PO Box 5488
Richmond, VA 23220-0488
AASECT@aasect.org

American Lung Association
1740 Broadway
New York, NY 10019
1-800-LUNG USA
212-315-8700
www.lungusa.org

American Massage Therapy
Association
820 Davis St.
Evanston, IL 60201
1-888-843-2682
www.amtamassage.org

American Music Therapy
Association

8455 Colesville Road
Suite 1000
Silver Spring, Maryland 20910
301-589-3300
www.musictherapy.org

American Transplant Association
980 North Michigan Avenue,
Suite 1400
Chicago, IL 60611
1-800-494-4527
ata@americantransplant.org

Canadian Lung Association
1900 City Park Drive, Suite 508
Blair Business Park
Gloucester, Ontario K1J 1A3
Canada

Cape COPD Support Group
c/o Clambake Celebrations
1223 Main Street
Chatham, MA 02633
A nonprofit support group.

Eldercare Locator
1-800-677-1116 (Monday–Friday,
9 A.M.–11 P.M. EST)
www.eldercare.gov

Family Caregiver Alliance
690 Market Street
Suite 600
San Francisco, CA 94104
415-434-3388
www.caregiver.org

Laughter Clubs
800-669-5233
614-855-4733 international
1159 South Creekway Ct.
Gahanna, Ohio 43230
www.laughterclubs.com

National Alliance for Caregiving
4720 Montgomery Lane
5th Floor
Bethesda, MD 20814
www.caregiving.org
A coalition of national not-for-profit
agencies

National Association for Home
Care
228 Seventh Street, SE
Washington, DC 20003
202-547-7424
www.nahc.org
This organization for home health
care agencies has a great deal of
helpful information, especially on
how to select a home care provider.

National Clearinghouse of
Rehabilitation Training Materials
1132 W. Hall of Fame
Oklahoma State University
Stillwater, OK 74078-4080
405-744-2000
800-223-2219
www.nchrtm.okstate.edu/index
3.html

National Emphysema Prevention
Program
www.nepp.org

National Emphysema/COPD
Association (NECA)
NECA
PO Box 11725
Kimberly Square Center
Albany, NY 12211-0725
www.NECACommunity.com
A relatively new nonprofit
organization whose mission is to
empower patients with emphysema

and COPD, as well as their families
and caregivers, to improve the quality
of their lives. A newsletter is
available.

National Family Caregivers
Association
10400 Connecticut Ave, #500
Kensington, MD 20895-3944
800-896-3650
www.nfcacares.org
A grass-roots organization created to
address the common needs and
concerns of all family caregivers.

National Heart, Lung, & Blood
Institute
301-592-8573
nhlbiinfo@rover.nhlbi.nih.gov
Ask for their book *Chronic
Obstructive Pulmonary Disease*, which
is available for $2. There is a
discounted rate for orders of twenty-
five or more copies.

National Jewish Medical and
Research Center
1400 Jackson Street
Denver, CO 80206
303-388-4461
1-800-222-LUNG (outside
Colorado) (8 A.M.–5 P.M. mountain
time)
303-398-1477 (within Colorado)
www.njc.org
Call to talk to a nurse or respiratory
therapist. Publishes newsletters *New
Directions* (for lay readers) and
Update (for physicians).

National Lung Health Education
Program
Health ONE Center

899 Logan Street
Denver, CO 80203-3130
nlhep@aol.com
www.nlhep.org

National Emphysema Foundation
15 Stevens Street
Norwalk, CT 06856
www.emphysemafoundation.org
gary@emphysemafoundation.org
Offers education and research
material.

Pulmonary Education & Research
Foundation
Second Wind Newsletter
PERF
PO Box 1133
Lomita, CA 90717-5133
310-539-8390
www.perf2ndwind.org

Society for Accessible Travel &
Hospitality (SATH)
347 Fifth Avenue, Suite 610
New York, NY 10016-4010
Tel: 212-447-7284
Fax: 212-725-8253
sathtravel@aol.com
www.sath.org
A nonprofit educational organization
offering worldwide listings of
accessible facilities including flights,
cruises, vans, hotels, and tourist
attractions.

Second Wind Lung Transplant
Association
300 South Duncan Ave., Suite 227
Clearwater, FL 33755-6457
888-855-9463 or 727-442-0892
www.2ndwind.org
heering@2ndwing.org

Visiting Nurses Association of America
PO Box 100697
Denver, CO 80250
800-426-2547
Check your telephone directory for your local health department to find the association nearest to you. There are more than 500 in the United States.

Well Spouse Foundation
63 West Main Street, Suite H
Freehold, NJ 07728
800-838-0879
www.wellspouse.org
An international, not-for-profit organization whose mission is to provide emotional support to, raise consciousness about, and advocate for the partners and children of the chronically ill and/or disabled. Newsletter and other information available.

www.http://familydoctor.org/handouts/003.html
This Web site has a myriad of medical information, including descriptions of advanced directives.

Harvard University School of Medicine
www.intelihealth.com
This Web site contains articles, basic fact sheets, and other information about COPD.

Mayo Clinic
www.mayoclinic.com
This prestigious site offers articles and other information that is of interest to those with COPD and their families.

National Library of Medicine
www.medlineplus.gov
This site offers an array of factual material including links to National Institutes of Health clearinghouses.

www.seniors.gov/articles/0301/advanced_directives.htm
This government site has information on numerous subjects of interest to seniors, including advance directives.

NOTE: Always check information at more than one Web site. As you check other health care Web sites, be sure you know who provided the information and when it was posted. Remember that Web sites sponsored by pharmaceutical companies may be biased towards their own products.

Resources to help you stop smoking

American Cancer Society
800-ACS-2345

American Heart Association
800-242-8721
Ask for their smoking packet.

American Lung Association
800-LUNG-USA

Centers for Disease Control
Office on Smoking and Health
800-311-3435
www.cdc.gov/tobacco/index.html

National Jewish Medical and
Research Center
800-222-LUNG
www.nationaljewish.org
Ask for their booklet, *Giving Up
Smoking.*

Nicotine Anonymous
Nicotine Anonymous World Services
419 Main Street, PMB #370
Huntington Beach, CA 92648
415-750-0328
www.nicotine-anonymous.org/

Words to Know

acute. Relatively brief, as opposed to chronic or long-lasting. A cold is an acute illness, whereas COPD is chronic.

ADE. Adverse drug event.

ADR. Adverse drug reaction.

alpha-1-antitrypsin (AAT). A material produced by the liver that protects the lungs against inflammation. A rare genetic defect sometimes prevents this enzyme from being produced, causing the individual to be more susceptible to COPD at an earlier age.

alveoli. Microscopic air sacs deep in the lungs where transfer of carbon dioxide from blood to the lungs and oxygen from air to the blood takes place.

anticholinergic. A medication, like Atrovent, used to open clogged bronchial tubes.

anti-inflammatory. A drug that fights inflammation. Drugs used to fight inflammation in the airways include Azmacort, Flovent, Pulmicort, and prednisone.

arterial blood gas analysis (ABG). A test in which blood is taken from an artery in your wrist to evaluate how effective your lungs are in bringing oxygen to the blood and removing carbon dioxide from it.

asthma. An acute inflammatory disease of the lungs in which the airways become swollen and filled with mucus.

asthmatic bronchitis. Inflammation of the bronchial tubes and smaller airways, causing a shortness of breath, a raspy throat, and coughing, often bringing up a lot of green or dark yellow sputum.

bacteria. Organisms that can cause infections such as chronic bronchitis.

beta$_2$-agonist. A type of drug that blocks or limits the effects of certain body chemicals that cause the airways to narrow. Beta$_2$-agonists allow the bronchial muscle tissue to relax and thus help open up the airways, especially the smaller airways. Examples of beta$_2$-agonists are Proventil, Ventolin, Serevent, and Alupent.

blebs and bullae. Destroyed portions of the lungs.

bronchi. Larger air passages of the lungs.

bronchial tubes. The two main airways that branch out from the windpipe, carrying air to the lungs.

bronchioles. Smallest branches of the bronchial tubes that lead to the lungs.

bronchodilator. Medication that relaxes the smooth muscles and opens constricted airways.

bronchospasm. A sudden contraction of the smooth muscle of the bronchi that causes an obstruction of the airway. It is distinguished by a cough and generalized wheezing.

capillaries. Microscopic blood vessels where oxygen and carbon dioxide are exchanged in the lungs.

carbon dioxide (CO_2). The waste product that passes out of the blood during breathing and is exhaled by the lungs.

catarrh. Inflammation of the mucous membranes causing a chronic cough and mucus discharge.

chronic. Long-standing illness, such as emphysema.

chronic obstructive lung disease (COLD). Another term for COPD.

cilia. Microscopic hairlike structures lining the airways. Their purpose is to wave bacteria, pollutants, and other materials upward where they can be expelled. In patients with COPD, these tiny hairs are destroyed and do not perform this function well or at all.

compliance. Following medical direction fully and correctly.

cor pulmonale. Enlargement of the heart's right ventricle caused by emphysema and chronic bronchitis.

corticosteroid. Steroid hormone like those made by the body's adrenal glands. In the form of inhaled medications, it is used to treat asthma and allergies.

cyanosis. Bluish color of the skin or nails associated with insufficient oxygen.

diaphragm. A large, curved, thin muscle dividing the chest from the abdominal cavity and used in breathing. When we inhale, the diaphragm flattens and sinks in order to help draw air into the lungs.

diuretic. Drug used to help the kidneys excrete salt and water.

DNR. Do not resuscitate. It is an order given by an individual or his or her health care surrogate that tells medical staff not to use heroic measures to restore consciousness or life

dyspnea. Shortness of breath.

edema. Swelling of the hands, arms, legs, and feet caused by retaining salt and water.

electrocardiogram (EKG). A noninvasive test measuring the heart's electrical activity.

emphysema. A disease in which the alveolar sacs in the lungs are enlarged or destroyed so they are no longer able to exchange oxygen from the air for waste gases in the bloodstream.

exacerbation. A period when a disease or medical condition gets worse. In chronic bronchitis, it's often due to a bacterial infection. The signs of an exacerbation include coughing more than usual, fever, and greenish or yellow sputum.

exertion. In the context of COPD, it means physical exertion, the act of using more energy than usual, such as in climbing stairs or walking fast.

exhalation. The act of breathing out.

expectorant. A substance used to thin out mucus secretions in the lungs.

forced expiratory volume (FEV). The volume of air that can be forcibly expelled quickly in one second after taking in a deep breath.

gas exchange. A primary function of the lungs involving transfer of oxygen from inhaled air to the blood and of carbon dioxide from the blood to the lungs.

gastroesophageal reflux disease (GERD). A disease in which stomach acid backs up into the esophagus, triggering a condition known as heartburn and, often, asthma.

genetic. Refers to heredity.

heartburn. A burning sensation in the chest caused by the regurgitation of stomach acid into the esophagus.

hypoventilation. A state in which too little air enters and leaves the lungs to bring oxygen into tissues and eliminate carbon dioxide.

hypoxemia. Not enough oxygen in the blood, caused by the inability of the alveoli in the lungs to properly exchange blood gases.

hypoxia. Reduced levels of oxygen in the tissues, often revealed by a blueish tint to the lips or fingernails.

immunosuppressant. Medication used to prevent the body from rejecting an organ transplant.

inflammation. The immune system's protective reaction to an irritant, such as your eyelid swelling when a bit of dust gets in your eye. Chronic inflammation usually involves formation of new connective tissue or a thickening, which can create problems. In COPD, it can make the airways narrower, making it more difficult for air to get through and for sputum to be coughed out.

inhalation. The act of breathing in. Also called inspiration.

inhaler. A device that helps a person breathe in medicine that goes directly to the lungs.

long-term oxygen therapy (LTOT). Using oxygen constantly for a lengthy period of time.

lymphatic. Refers to the lymph system, the part of the body's immune system that makes white blood cells, which fight infection.

macrophage. Scavenger cells in the lungs that carry away irritants.

maintenance. Continuing on a long-term or permanent basis, as in maintenance therapy.

metered-dose inhaler (MDI). A device that dispenses a fixed dosage of medication through an inhaler.

mucus. A thick liquid that moistens and lubricates body tissues, including those in the airways and lungs.

nebulizer. A device for making a spray, like an atomizer. Medicines for COPD may be delivered in this manner by projecting the medication through a mask worn by the patient.

nicotine. The addictive substance in tobacco.

nicotine-replacement products. Medications that contain nicotine, generally in the form of gum, a skin patch, or an inhaler, that are used to decrease the discomfort of withdrawal from smoking. Some are now available over-the-counter while others still require a doctor's prescription.

over-the-counter (OTC). Refers to medications that are available at your pharmacy without a prescription.

oxygen (O_2). The most important component in air, an element essential for life, which enters the bloodstream through the lungs.

pack-year. A measure of someone's cigarette smoking over a lifetime: the number of packs per day times the number of years a person has smoked. In other words, ten pack-years could refer to a smoking history of two packs a day for five years, one pack a day for ten years, or half a pack a day for twenty years.

peak flow meter. A device that measures the rate at which a person can exhale.

percussing. Tapping your back in order to hear the sound of air density.

peripheral edema. Swelling in the ankles or legs signifying fluid retention, a possible sign of heart complications.

phlegm. Thick, sticky substances produced by the respiratory tract, usually as the result of irritation, inflammation, or infection of the airways. Also called sputum or mucus.

pleura. A thin membrane encasing the lungs and lining the chest cavity.

prophylactic treatment. Therapy used to prevent an illness or symptom from developing.

pulmonary. Having to do with the lungs.

pulmonary function test (PFT). Test used to determine lung function.

pulmonologist. A physician who specializes in treating diseases of the lungs.

pulse oximetry. A device, usually clipped onto a finger or the ear, used for measuring the amount of oxygen in the blood.

pursed-lips breathing. A technique used by those with COPD, in which air is inhaled slowly through the nose and mouth and then exhaled slowly through pursed lips. The purpose is to control shortness of breath.

rale. Breath sounds that may suggest lung problems such as asthma, pneumonia, or emphysema.

red blood cells. Blood cells containing hemoglobin that transport oxygen to tissues.

reflux. The backward flow of stomach acid into the esophagus. Commonly known as heartburn.

rescue medication. A short-acting medication designed to relieve breathing difficulty symptoms quickly.

respiration. Taking air into the lungs, then exhaling it. Another word for breathing.

respiratory tract. The entire system of organs and tissues involved in breathing: especially the lungs, trachea, bronchial tubes, bronchioles, and alveoli.

S.O.B. Shortness of breath.

spirometer. A device into which one blows (exhales quickly) to measure breathing capacity.

sputum. *See phlegm.*

thorax. The chest.

trachea. The tube leading from the vocal cords to the area of the lungs, where it divides into the two main bronchi. Also called windpipe.

virus. An organism that can cause a wide variety of infections, including colds and the flu. Antibiotics are not effective against viruses, although they are sometimes given to prevent secondary infections.

wheeze. A specific sound in breathing caused by air being forced through mucus and a narrowed airway.

white blood cells. Cells that fight infection and allergies. Also called leukocytes.

Suggested Reading

Benson, Herbert, M.D., with Miriam Z. Klipper. *The Relaxation Response.* New York: Avon Books, 1975.

Benson, Herbert, M.D., with Marg Stark. *Timeless Healing: The Power and Biology of Belief.* New York: Scribner, 1996.

Blau, Sheldon P., M.D., F.A.C.P., F.A.C.R., and Elaine Fantle Shimberg. *How to Get Out of the Hospital Alive.* New York: Macmillan, 1997.

Carter, Rosalynn. *Helping Yourself Help Others.* New York: Times Books, 1994.

Carter, Rick, Ph.D., Brooke Nicotra, M.D., and Jo Von Tucker. *Courage and Information for Life with Chronic Obstructive Pulmonary Disease.* Onset, MA: New Technology Publishing, 2001.

Cousins, Norman. *Anatomy of an Illness.* New York: Bantam, 1981.

Goldfarb, Lori A., Mary Jane Brotherson, Jean Ann Summers, and Ann P. Turnbull. *Meeting the Challenge of Disability or Chronic Illness—A Family Guide.* Baltimore: Paul H. Brookes, 1986.

Good, James T., Jr., M.D., and Thomas L. Petty, M.D. *Frontline Advice for COPD Patients.* Denver: Snowdrift Pulmonary Conference, 2002.

Grollman, Earl A. *Caring and Coping When Your Loved One is Seriously Ill.* Boston: Beacon Press, 1995.

Haas, Francois, and Sheila Sperber Haas. *The Chronic Bronchitis and Emphysema Handbook.* New York: John Wiley & Sons, Inc., 2000.

Heymann, Jody, M.D. *Equal Partners.* Philadelphia: University of Pennsylvania Press, 2000.

Jenkins, Mark. *Chronic Obstructive Pulmonary Disease: Practical Medical and Spiritual Guidelines for Daily Living with Emphysema, Chronic Bronchitis & Combination Diagnosis* Center City, MN: Hazelden Information Education, 1999.

Leahey, Maureen R.N., Ph.D., and Lorraine M. Wright, R.N., Ph.D. *Families & Life-Threatening Illness*. Springhouse, PA: Springhouse Corporation, 1987.

Moos, Rudolf H., ed. *Coping with Physical Illness*. New York: Plenum, 1984.

National Heart, Lung, & Blood Institute. *Chronic Obstructive Pulmonary Disease*: PO Box 30105, Bethesda, MD 20824-0105; 301-592-8573.

Oster, Nancy, Lucy Thomas, and Darol Joseff, M.D. *Making Informed Medical Decisions*. Sebastopol, CA: O'Reilly & Associates, 2000.

Petty, Thomas L., M.D., and Dennis E. Doherty, M.D. *Save Your Breath, America! Advice for Patients Who May Be Developing Emphysema or Chronic Bronchitis* Thomas L. Petty, M.D., 1850 High Street, Denver, CO 80218.

Petty, Thomas L., M.D., and Louise M. Nett. *Enjoying Life with Chronic Obstructive Pulmonary Disease*. Cedar Grove, NJ: Laennec Publishing, 1995.

Register, Cheri. *Living with Chronic Illness*. New York: Macmillan, 1987.

Rolland, John S., M.D. *Families, Illness, & Disability*. New York: Basic Books, 1994.

Shapiro, Howard M. *Dr. Shapiro's Picture Perfect Weight Loss*. Emmaus, PA: Rodale, 2000.

Siegel, Bernie S., M.D. *Love, Medicine & Miracles*. New York: Harper, 1986.

Weil, Andrew, M.D. *Natural Health, Natural Medicine*. Boston: Houghton Mifflin, 1995.

Yeager, Selene, and Bridget Doherty. *The Prevention Get Thin, Get Young Plan*. Emmaus, PA: Rodale, 2001.

Zilbergeld, Bernie, Ph.D., and Arnold Lazarus, Ph.D. *Mind Power: Getting What You Want Through Mental Training*. Boston: Little, Brown, 1987.

Index

About the Author

Elaine Fantle Shimberg is an award-winning medical writer of books about depression, strokes, Tourette syndrome, irritable bowel syndrome, chronic heartburn (acid reflux or GERD), and other conditions. She is the first layperson to serve on the Florida Medical Association's Ethical and Judicial Affairs Committee, is past president of the Florida chapter of the American Medical Writers Association, and is chairman of the board of St. Joseph's-Baptist Hospital in the Tampa Bay area. Recently, she received an honorary doctor of humane letters degree from the University of South Florida. Shimberg divides her time between Scarborough, Maine, and Tampa, Florida.